Contents

v

Preface

A preface *and* an introduction may seem an editorial indulgence. Even an introduction alone is a luxury. We have felt, none the less, that each is in this case desirable – the latter to help draw this collection of essays together by identifying their common threads, and the former – this preface – to set out the authors' intentions and to avert possible misunderstanding about the nature of the exercise attempted here.

Firstly, it has been the authors' intention to reach as wide an audience as possible, since the problems of the health service are of great interest to many people. Thus, while all of us are economists, we have either avoided the use of technical terms or, where necessary, attempted to explain them.

Secondly, it has been the authors' intention to avoid policy conclusions – both final and even tentative conclusions. Instead we have tried to show how our branch of social science can shed light on some key questions about the National Health Service, and thereby help people to make up their minds about some of the great issues that confront us; issues that include questions about the aims of the Service and how it should be financed. While we all undoubtedly have views about how policy should be shaped, these views are at least as much influenced by our personal value systems as they are formed by our professional knowledge. It is the latter in which we claim a special competence and it is only the latter, therefore, that we believe should be given prominence in a collection such as this.

We have been encouraged in our self-denial by the Royal Commission on the National Health Service, whose interpretation of their terms of reference in *The Task Ahead* identified sixty explicit topics relating to its general intention, in its own words, 'to ask fundamental questions about the NHS'. As an indicator of how fundamental they were prepared to be, the first issue identified was 'what is meant by "health"'. The answers to questions such as this were seen by the Commission as essential background to their ultimate tasks of evaluating NHS policy and making policy recommendations. In this approach they are surely correct.

Nevertheless, we confidently predict our attempt at a relatively impartial discussion of (some of) the issues will stand out as unusual among the welter of partisan publishing that will precede, accompany and succeed the Commission's report. In this respect the admirable example set by the Commission will be followed by very few. Neither do we doubt that we ourselves shall be accused by some (a minority, we hope) of cowardice in the face of the policy issues and by others (equally a minority, we hope) of secretly infiltrating our own insidious values on an unsuspecting and gullible public. Our only defence will be that we have sincerely tried to contribute that which we have a special competence to contribute – so our intentions are pure. It is for the reader to judge our success.

Contributors

J. A. CAIRNS is a Research Fellow at the Institute of Social and Economic Research at York.

A. J. CULYER is a Reader in Economics and Assistant Director of the Institute of Social and Economic Research at York.

M. F. DRUMMOND is a Research Fellow at the Institute of Social and Economic Research at York.

R. J. LAVERS is a Research Fellow at the Institute of Social and Economic Research at York.

A. K. MAYNARD is a Senior Lecturer in Economics at the University of York.

M. C. SNELL is a Research Fellow at the Institute of Social and Economic Research at York.

A. WALKER is a Research Fellow at the Institute of Social and Economic Research at York.

A. WILLIAMS is a Professor of Economics at the University of York.

K. G. WRIGHT is a Senior Research Fellow at the Institute of Social and Economic Research at York.

ACKNOWLEDGEMENTS

Most of the chapters in this volume have benefited from comments made on them by all the people listed above and, therefore, each author wishes to acknowledge the help he has received from the others. Acknowledgements to other people who have commented on papers are included in the footnotes to each paper.

1. Introduction

A. J. Culyer and K. G. Wright

The essays in this volume are all concerned with aspects of the central issue occupying economists – the issue of *choice*. How are choices made? How *ought* choices to be made? What consequences will follow from particular choices? How may changes in the decision-making environment affect choices? The necessity of choice arises partly because some of the ends sought by man are mutually inconsistent, and partly – which is the central core of economics – because the means by which the ends may be achieved are strictly limited by resource constraints and by rules defining (and hence limiting) the uses to which scarce resources may be put. While there are some who deny the real scarcity of resources, and blame the problems of the National Health Service (NHS) on the unions, capitalism, bureaucrats or whatever, and still others who look confidently ahead to an age when either technology will have abolished scarcity or, alternatively, men's wants will have become sufficiently modest that scarcity will no longer have relevance, we take the view that the economic problems of making the 'best' use of our resources exist independently of the social arrangements adopted for their solution and, in any case, are not in immediate prospect of disappearance as far as Britain's National Health Service is concerned.

The real problem arises in trying to define what is 'best use'. As far as health is concerned, one line of thought is offered by the Royal Commission's terms of reference 'to consider in the interests both of the patients and of those who work in the National Health Service the best use and management of the financial and manpower resources of the National Health Service' (Royal Commission on the NHS, 1976, p. 1). This is, however, a narrower concern than that of the economist, who is usually concerned with the maximisation of the net benefit of the community as a whole, rather than the benefit of particular sub-groups of producers and consumers. Nevertheless, the way in which this benefit is most appropriately measured, and the determination of whose judgements are to be incorporated, remains a central theme of the book.

1

There are several reasons for supposing that leaving choices in health care to private individuals alone (doctors, nurses, patients, owners, administrators, etc.) would result in an outcome that would generally be agreed to be unsatisfactory. These reasons, arising from inherent characteristics of choice in health care (and giving rise to questions of profound philosophical difficulty and policy importance) are basically three.

(i) There is an asymmetry in the amount of information available to the various contracting parties. In particular, the supplier of service not only has more technical knowledge than the client, but he is also employed as adviser to the client as to which services ought to be received. Moreover, as supplier, the physician makes decisions concerning very valuable resources (on average, a consultant allocates resources roughly valued at £250,000 per annum (Owen, 1976)), of which he himself is not the owner. As guardian of the patient's interests he therefore plays his traditional role, but *quis custodiet custodies*? Who, precisely, makes what choices? What would follow from some alteration in the parameters of these choices? Who should evaluate whose needs and within what resources constraints? Who should decide these constraints?

(ii) The individual is often uncertain about the effects of the choices open to him. He may not know anything about the costs that treatment will impose on him and he may not be able to judge the quality of the care that is given to him. For both this and the first reason individuals have good reason to 'consult' a doctor. But, it turns out, doctors too are extremely uncertain about the effects of their choices or, where certain, they may nevertheless be simply wrong (Cochrane, 1972). What incentives exist in the system to discourage inefficient decisions by patients and doctors and to reduce uncertainty? How far should one pursue preventive programmes? How far should one monitor and control professional and clinical decision-making? How far should abuse by patients be tolerated? What *is* patient abuse?

(iii) An individual's health is of concern to other people as well as himself. This concern for others may be motivated by altruism. Some people may be concerned about other people's health and seek to help or ensure that help is available to the sick. Attitudes to others may be motivated by more selfish concern. As more people are immunised against an infectious disease, the risk of contracting it is lowered for those who have not been immunised. In addition, it may well be worth while for those who are well to support the provision of facilities for the treatment of people who are currently ill, because doing so creates the capacity that may be needed to treat those who are well now but may be ill in the future. Finally, and by no means least, modern societies seem to be preoccupied with the income-distributional problems that may arise in connection with health care expenditures. How, then, are these 'external' effects to be measured? And how is their existence to be taken into account in the choices that are made? Are there any limits to the collective intervention that these concerns suggest may be desirable?

These three reasons would seem to lie at the root of many of the economic problems of health services. Many would claim that the answers to the questions to which they give rise provide the fundamental case for having a national health service. If this is the case then no important discussion of health policy – let alone an economic discussion of the NHS – can avoid broaching the question of the meaning, relevance and operationality of the concept of 'need'. Nor can such a discussion evade matters of evaluating the methods and procedures adopted in the clinical practice of medicine. Nor, finally, can such a discussion evade the problems raised by the existence of third-party interests with a legitimate (or so it is asserted) claim upon the attention of those whose values will determine policy.

Moreover, once the legitimacy of a *collective* interest in the provision of health services is granted, then further questions immediately come to the fore. In particular, we have an important set of problems concerned with the policy-making itself. This process may be seen as a series of steps:

(i) the identification of the problems to be found over the next ten or so years;
(ii) the definition of objectives to tackle the problems identified;
(iii) the identification of alternative ways of achieving those objectives;
(iv) the analysis of the effects of these alternatives;
(v) taking decisions in the light of this analysis;
(vi) monitoring the effectiveness of policy in meeting the stated objectives and taking any necessary corrective action.

Economics has a central role in the analysis of the three characteristics discussed above, not least because inferences drawn from them seem to erode substantially any presumption that health services can be treated as a *laissez-faire* sector of social life. Economics is also crucial in most of the six policy-making steps. Of course, the present volume cannot cover all the questions facing the NHS, but each of the contributions can be clearly seen as a member of the economic family, and between them they cover a reasonable range of problems to which economists in the health territory have addressed themselves. To maximise the range, contributors have, where the topic allowed and the material existed, presented synoptic *reviews* of arguments, derived results (both conceptual and empirical), and offered some assessment of the present state of the art.

The book has grown up around evidence submitted by some of us to the Royal Commission on the National Health Service in the belief that economics has a useful part to play in helping people to make up their minds about some of the issues confronting policy-makers in the NHS. Those contributing have sought no unifying theme, or 'attitude', in their contributions other than that provided anyway by an economic approach. Indeed, we have resisted the temptation to present any set of final 'answers' to or resolutions of policy questions. By contrast we have actively focused our attention on the 'questions', in the belief both that satisfactory answers are not to be found to unsatisfactory questions and that economics as a method of analysis is particularly helpful in the formulation of relevant questions.

However, we have not been concerned solely with the questions, for a distinctive if subsidiary characteristic of the economic analysis is its ability to analyse different approaches to answering questions with the intention of setting out the issues involved in a manner that is helpful for decision-making but that carefully avoids making specific policy recommendations. We can illustrate the approach from the chapter by Cairns and Snell on pricing (Chapter 7), in which they focus explicitly and in detail on the questions: 'What effect is charging prices likely to have on the demand for health services and how do we set about evaluating different pricing policies?' and 'What effects does experience tell us they have actually had?' Having theorised, provided a framework for evaluation and identified the known relevant facts, it is left to the reader to form his own conclusions in the light of his own values and experience. Thus the authors do not themselves presume to judge the desirability of charging prices for health care. This self-denial is still a minority characteristic, even among academic students of health services, let alone those with particular axes to grind. Among the many (certainly hundreds) of articles to have appeared in Britain during the last decade concerning the issue of charges or prices, the ratio of analysis and evidence to pure exhortation and deliberate persuasion is very small. Far too frequently there has been, and not only among social scientists, a refusal to distinguish between the advancement of knowledge and the promotion of policy – with the former often subordinated to the latter.

In view of the comments just made about the way social scientists have treated health service problems, those who are less familiar with the literature might be forgiven for expecting that it consists largely of philosophical, *a priori*, discussion whereby policy inferences are eventually drawn from first principles. Far from it. The way in which health 'needs' have been discussed epitomises the shallowness of much of the discussion and its methodological unsophistication. It has been shallow and unsophisticated in several ways. At its crudest, 'needs' have been asserted with the corollary, either explicit or (more usually) implicit, that they must be met (regardless, of course, of cost). This gives rise to a second characteristic economic approach which concerns itself less with theory or facts as such than with the fundamental conceptual *mode of thought* to be adopted – in this case with respect to the notion of 'need'. The crucial questions about 'need', to which Williams, Wright and Culyer attempt in Part I to lend a more precise and operational formulation, were (almost) invariably left unanswered: Who decides what is needed (what criteria are used to select the 'who', and what criteria do the 'who' in turn use to select the 'needs'?); how does 'need' relate to other notions such as 'demand'; how can 'need' be measured, compared with other 'needs', compared with 'cost'?

While these criticisms are perhaps in a small degree less valid today than they were five years ago – credit for which phenomenon must at least in part be given to economists and other students of health services with economics or related backgrounds – the methodology from which they derive retains its validity in full.

Thus, in summary, the present collection represents these two kinds of characteristic approach, the first exploring both the theoretical and empirical consequences of choices and actions; the second exploring the logical nature of the choices that have to be made and developing a language and conceptual framework that may be helpful in setting out the problems. The technical skills – such as they are – of economists do not permit them to go any further. But we trust that they may help others to go further – in particular, we trust that they may help in the development of rational and humane social policies in the health territory. To reiterate, the presentation of material in this way is intended to help people to make up their own minds on the basis of the contributors' accounts of what a great many experts have thought about, concluded, and discovered in the way of facts. We most emphatically do not intend to make up anyone's mind for him.

REFERENCES

Cochrane, A. L. (1972) *Effectiveness and Efficiency: Random Reflections on Health Services* London, Nuffield Provincial Hospitals Trust.

Owen, David (1976) 'Clinical Freedom and Professional Freedom' *The Lancet* 8 May 1976, pp. 1006–9.

Royal Commission on the National Health Service (1976) *The Task Ahead* London, HMSO.

PART I

Quality of Care

2. Need, Values and Health Status Measurement

A. J. Culyer[1]

Although it has become fashionable for some economists to take the (or rather, an) idea of 'need' seriously, and for them to urge others (such as royal commissioners) also to take it seriously, it takes little in the way of a literature search before one realises that the path, though not much trodden by social scientists, resembles more of a beaten track from other perspectives. The idea of this chapter is to link the rather broad exegetical work of Williams with the detailed empirical work of Wright (examples of both of which are in the present volume) and in so doing both to attempt to show how need, (some) values, and the frequently highly technical issues in health status measurement involve interlinked ideas, and to illustrate the linkages from a highly selected sample of empirical work performed by operations researchers and researchers in clinical medicine.

Although I shall be highly selective in what is drawn from a large and disparate literature, the objective is openly to be both persuasive and pedagogic: to persuade others of the immense importance of the work being undertaken and of its centrality to the issues involved in planning health services to meet people's needs as best as possible; and to introduce those who may not be familiar with it to some of the hard empirical work that has been done while providing an intellectually 'whole' context in which this work may be best interpreted.

2.1 DEFINITION OF 'NEED'

A definition, while conducive to clear understanding, has the disadvantage of placing its author clearly in the line of fire. The definition proffered here is followed by a brief discussion of some implications and some acknowledged limitations.

A need for health care exists when:

(i)   the potential for *avoidance* of reductions in health status exists (prevention and some care);
(ii) the potential for *improvements* in health status above the level it would otherwise be exists (cure and some care).[2]

Implicit in this definition is the proposition that the health services exist to minimise need or, what is the same thing, to effect the maximum increase in the health status of the client population, in each case subject to the important limitation 'given the resources available'.

Using Williams's terminology, the definition is a 'quasi-supply' concept: a need exists only if a procedure has a positive expected outcome. Yet it also has, as we shall shortly see, important 'demand'-type attributes. These are inherent because the relationships between 'procedures' and 'outcomes' defined in terms of health status are not, and cannot be, only technological – as seems to be implied by the quasi-supply notion. The concept of health status is heavily imbued with values and trade-offs of a subjective nature, indeed of precisely the nature normally considered in economic discussion of 'demand', so that no neat distinction can properly be drawn between 'supply' and 'demand' in the medical sphere. It is, of course, well known that the traditional dichotomy between these two breaks down in other respects: for example, the normal equilibrating properties of demand and supply are highly attenuated, if not wholly destroyed, by the role of the physician as an agent for his clients; he largely determines both what they shall demand and what will be supplied (see Chapter 7 below). This is yet another instance of the peculiar (at least to economists!) nature of health care. 'Need' is thus simultaneously a quasi-supply and a quasi-demand concept.

An unfortunate feature of the definition as presented is that it excludes the possibility of a need for care that may have no impact upon health status but may be comforting to patients, particularly those with terminal illness or chronic conditions whose natural history has little possibility of alteration but where the provision of 'loving care' may be legitimately regarded as being 'needed'. This is an issue that we set aside for the moment, not on the grounds that it is unimportant or likely to become less important (quite the contrary!), nor on the grounds that the framework adopted here could not be adjusted to incorporate it, but simply for the reason that doing the latter is a job for subsequent consideration and that, for the moment, we have quite enough on our plates as it is.

The related implication, that there can be no need where there is no currently available and effective procedure, is not, however, merely a question of the order in which we tackle problems. It is, rather, an important feature of the definition. Plainly, it is not meaningless in general to speak about someone needing a treatment that does not (as yet) exist. But our definition, in excluding such a connotation, is less limiting than may appear, for the 'potential' for affecting health status now attaches itself by implication to the prospects for *research* rather than prevention, cure or care. That is, those who are seen as needing non-existent treatments are best seen as in need of the results of successfully prosecuted research. This would seem also to focus policy thinking in the right direction.

Finally, the definition does *not* imply that need is an absolute – to be met, for example, regardless of other needs, or to be met regardless of cost.[3] The fact that a 'potential' may *exist* does not imply that it should be *realised*, for realising a potential uses up resources that could have been put to other desired ends, and a balance must be struck. Indeed, if one adopts the view that the proper general objective of the NHS is to maximise the impact of the nation's chosen allocation to the NHS upon health needs (as is the view in Culyer, 1976), then it follows that marginal needs will remain unmet.[4] The comforting corollary is that they will be, out of those needs capable technically of being met, the most trivial in social terms per unit of resource.

With this definition and its corollaries in mind, we turn in the rest of the chapter to the place of values in health status measurement. In particular, we focus upon three kinds of value judgement: the choice of dimensions in which health status is to be measured; the choice of weights by which various dimensions are to be 'traded off', and the choice of numbers to be assigned to the dimensions that have, in this way, been combined.[5]

2.2 VALUES AND HEALTH STATUS

2.2.1 Dimensions

Not all the judgements that have to be made are value judgements. This is important to recognise, since the qualifications persons are required to have to make judgements of fact or judgements about technology need not be the same as the qualifications they are required to have to make judgements of value. Such an observation may appear *jejune* and uncontroversial. Nevertheless, at least one distinguished economist would dissent from it:

My personal feeling is that the value-judgements made by economists are, by and large, better than those made by non-economists! ... My assertion about value judgements is not as arrogant as it sounds. For one thing, it applies only to the sort of value-judgements involved in public investment decisions, and even here does not apply to all of them.... The point is simply that the people who are experienced at systematic thinking about a problem are usually those who make the best judgements about it. Thus, whatever their theory of aesthetics, most people are prepared in practice to accept the judgement of an art critic about the merits of a painting. [Turvey, 1963, p. 96]

Unfortunately it is not clear from this, or from the example (not quoted) Turvey gives, which value judgements actually are best made by economists or, more generally, by 'experts'. Nor is it clear why 'systematic thinking' (presumably referring to the kind of thoughts characteristically had by economists) is conducive to 'good' value judgements – though we may readily concede that economists (or any systematic thinkers) may be quite adept at distinguishing value judgements from other kinds of judgement. Indeed, such distinctions are what we may reasonably expect from systematic thought of any kind.

One distinguished sociologist has made the point very forcibly with regard to the autonomy of the medical profession:

There is a real danger of a new tyranny which sincerely expresses itself in the language of humanitarianism and which imposes its own values on others for what it sees to be their own good.... [We should be concerned with] delineating the question of what is expertise and what concealed class morality, and what is actual performance rather than unrealizable ethical intent.... It is my own opinion that the professions' role in a free society should be limited to contributing the technical information men need to make their own decisions on the basis of their own values. When he preempts the authority to direct, even constrain men's decisions on the basis of his own values, the professional is no longer an expert but rather a member of a new privileged class disguised as an expert. [Freidson, 1970, pp. 381–2]

The value judgements we shall discuss here are arguably 'best' (i.e. legitimately) made by non-experts – in particular by non-economists *and* by non-physicians. As far as choice of dimensions is concerned, however, part of the selection can be made quite independently of value judgements: the judgements that are required are of quite different kinds.

Some of these points can be illustrated from the well worked territory of programmes designed to help the elderly. The objectives of such programmes are commonly defined in rather broad terms such as social integration (to reduce social isolation of the elderly within the community); self-dependence (to preserve identity and independence of the elderly); physical wellbeing (Algie, 1972). These aspirations are, of course, essential value judgements; and, although the experience of social workers may be helpful in identifying different ways of, say, integrating such people, and that of economists in costing alternative procedures, the value systems implying that these dimensions are, or should be, the objectives of policy do not necessarily emanate from, or only from, such professional groups.

By contrast, from the *circumstances* of the case it may sometimes be inferred that some specific dimensions are more relevant than others. Thus, a programme where the physical abilities of elderly persons in residential homes are thought relevant would not normally be concerned with ability to cook, do shopping or carpet cleaning because such tasks are not performed by such persons (Wright, 1974). The *purpose* of the exercise likewise may suggest some measures of ability as being more relevant than others: ability to cut toenails may be an important component in an indicator of the need for chiropody services, but there may be superior indicators measuring the impact of a programme on patients' general ability to manage for themselves: ability to dress measures ability to grasp and manipulate small objects (zips, buttons, etc.), to bend and stretch, etc. Clearly, there may also exist correlations between abilities enabling some to be eliminated as redundant in an index of general physical wellbeing. Such analysis is largely value-free. For reasons such as these Wright (in Chapter 4 below) eliminated some skills from his self-care schedule without implying in any way that the eliminated skills are 'unimportant' in a personal or social sense.

It is sometimes the case that a 'lexicographic' ordering of characteristics adequately scales a continuum of sickness or disability which obviates the necessity for trading off the individual characteristics. For example, if individuals having difficulty with feeding also have difficulty with continence, ambulation, dressing and bathing, and individuals having difficulty with continence also have difficulty with ambulation, dressing and bathing (but not with feeding), and individuals having difficulty with ambulation also have difficulty with dressing and bathing, etc. (but not with feeding and continence), then for the above five characteristics each dichotomised into difficulty/no difficulty states, the potential 2^5 ($= 32$) combinations can be collapsed into six categories of degrees of dependence as indicated in table 2.1. The scale (or order) is termed a 'Guttman scale' (after Guttman, 1944), and whether it is possible or useful depends, of course, in part on the combinations of patient states that are actually observed. Thus, if as many patients have (Yes, No, No, No, No) as (No, No, No, No, Yes), the scale will not be of much help. The better the 'fit' in this sense, the more perfect the scale type. How perfect one requires it to be is a matter largely of judgement.

TABLE 2.1
Guttman Scale of Patient Dependence

Degree of dependence	Feeding	Continence	Ambulation	Dressing	Bathing
1	No	No	No	No	No
2	No	No	No	No	Yes
3	No	No	No	Yes	Yes
4	No	No	Yes	Yes	Yes
5	No	Yes	Yes	Yes	Yes
6	Yes	Yes	Yes	Yes	Yes

There exist methods of adjusting characteristics and the cut-off points that determine whether a 'yes' or a 'no' answer is recorded that maximise the 'perfection' of the Guttman scale (Tenhouten, 1969), and which were utilised by Skinner and Yett (1973) to derive a Guttman scale of debility for patients needing skilled nursing care in a cost study of nursing homes. The technique, where applicable, has an obvious use as an ordinal indicator of 'need'. Skinner and Yett (1973) were able to identify the distribution of patients

TABLE 2.2

Percentage distribution of 21,036 patients by degree of dependence

Location	Degree of dependence					
	1	2	3	4	5	6
Nursing homes	14.9	12.0	24.5	12.2	12.1	24.3
Long-term hospital	23.0	10.3	19.1	13.5	12.8	21.3
Long-term unit in general hospital	23.0	10.8	16.2	17.3	12.6	20.1

Source: Skinner and Yett (1973), p. 75.

by dependence and institution as in table 2.2. It should be noted that the categories they used were those developed by Katz *et al.* (1963) in devising their index of activities of daily living for elderly persons with fractured hips. This pioneering work used dichotomous yes/no categories and devised an ordinal index, where the states are merely ranked in order of severity as follows:

A   independent in feeding, continence, transferring, going to toilet, dressing, and bathing
B   independent in all but one of these functions
C   independent in all but bathing and one additional function
D   independent in all but bathing, dressing and one additional function
E   independent in all but bathing, dressing, going to toilet and one additional function
F   independent in all but bathing, dressing, going to toilet, transferring and one additional function
G   dependent in all six functions
Other   dependent in at least two functions, but not classifiable as C, D, E or F

In the further sample of 1001 old persons (not necessarily with fracture of the hip) only 4 per cent fell into the 'Other' category, and it seems clear that this procedure is an extremely effective one for these categories in deriving an ordinal index of dependence. The dichotomous nature of the units of measuring ability to function, however, has been criticised by several authors (Wright, 1974 and references there) and makes the approach inappropriate where focus is upon degrees of dependency of a subtler kind. Its usefulness has been proved, however, in prognosis where it enables the avoidance of prolonged therapeutic efforts whose outcome, as measured by the index, is unlikely to be successful.

Another statistical technique that has been used is factor analysis. Levine and Yett (1973) used this in order to reduce a large number of regional indicators of health status, environment and socioeconomic conditions into a more manageable number of variables (four in their case). The essence of the procedure is to hypothesise that there exists some variable 'health status' that is a function of a smaller set of unobservable *factors* which underly the sixty-three (in their case) available indicators. The idea is to derive weights or 'loadings' based on the correlation between observed variables such that the factors are uncorrelated with one another while the loadings are regression coefficients of factors that explain a high proportion of the variance of the *j*th observed indicator. By observing the factor with the highest loading for each observed variable, the latter may then be grouped into clusters that (hopefully) make sense (e.g., all observed variables concerning income have relatively high loadings on one factor). For each cluster a composite index is then derived statistically and these can be related to social, demographic and economic variables.

This technique has been of use in some areas (e.g. psychology) where there is little theory available to determine which variables are or ought to be relevant and there may be some use for it in value-free applications in the health territory; for example, in ascertaining what variables or groups of variables have greatest impact on mortality. Since, however, nothing of normative import can be inferred from an analysis making no normative assumptions, and since normative issues largely predominate in status measurement (what is 'need'? Is that disability 'worse' than this one? Is a sick child 'worth' priority over an equally sick adult?), we propose no further discussions of factor analysis here. The procedure would seem *not* to be appropriate for the purpose conceived for it by Levine and Yett, namely, to identify areas whose health status is low. Low health status is a policy issue that cannot be resolved on grounds of correlation alone. And this quite aside from the inherent abstruseness of a technique, which is scarcely likely to commend itself for this if no other reason to the political masters, administrative managers and clinical practitioners in health services. This must especially be the case since nobody is proposing that health status measures should wholly supplant professional, political and administrative judgement. The aim is to *supplement* these informal judgements in order to make social judgements more systematically. It therefore follows that too high a degree of sophistication, producing results that are hard to interpret, is absolutely to be avoided.

We thus find that choice of the dimensions of an index is partly a question of values, of interpreting the specific objects of policy, and partly a technical question, concerning valid, reliable, economical and reproducible methods of measuring the objects. Just as persons who may legitimately be thought to have a claim on the right to formulate objects of policy (e.g. the elderly, the representatives of those financing the programme) may have little competence in deciding those matters we have described as 'technical', so those with this latter competence are not necessarily those regarded as having a legitimate right to decide objectives, or dimensions of indexes.

2.2.2   Weights

For evaluative purposes, the necessity for trade-offs will normally be inescapable even to identify only the qualitative direction of change in an individual's or a group's condition, a matter discussed at some length in Chapter 4. Precisely the same weighting problem arises in connection with geographical comparisons between areas and with longitudinal trends where an overall view is required, regardless of whether it is related to procedures, environment changes or medical interventions.

Miller (1970) identifies essentially the same problem in ranking the social impact of various diseases, where the ranking is quite different depending on whether inpatient days, outpatient visits or deaths is used and, hence, quite different priorities for programme expenditures are implied. He developed the 'Q index' for the US Indian Health Service, which is proposed as just one tool for management in deciding programme priorities, and which combined consideration of mortality and morbidity into a single index:

$$Q = (M_i/M_a)DP + \frac{(274A + 91.3B)}{N}$$

where

M_i = age- and sex-adjusted mortality rate of the Indian population;
M_a = age- and sex-adjusted mortality rate of the total US population;
D = crude mortality rate of Indian population;
P = years of life lost because of premature death in the Indian population (*viz.* the difference between average age of death among Indians and among US population as a whole);
A = hospital days in Indian population;
B = outpatient visits in Indian population;
N = Indian population.

The Q index is clearly a *relative* concept measuring Indian health status relative to that of the US population as a whole, though as Chen (1973) pointed out it is odd that the morbidity elements (A and B) are not made relative. Indeed, Chen made a number of suggestions for improving this index which we will briefly look at below. Here let us pause to note some of the weights that are applied in the Q index. First, A and B are weighted to convert them to years per 100,000 population with three outpatient visits equated in time to one hospital day (since it takes the average Indian one-third of a day to obtain outpatient care, including travel time). The implication of this is that, for a given disease (if the Q index is computed by disease category), the amount of time spent receiving care is the only relevant distinguishing characteristic. The fact (if it *is* a fact!) that hospitalised cases may be more serious cases than outpatient cases is not given weight. It may, of course, be replied that the idea of the Q index is to use currently available data only and to keep the index as straightforward as possible. Against this one might argue that it is no more complex conceptually or practically to weight A and B according to some judgements of their relative seriousness than it is to find out how much more time the one uses up relative to the other. Second, the simple addition of the mortality and the morbidity terms clearly begs many questions. While it would doubtless be claimed that the absence of data precludes more sophisticated weightings, against this it may again be said that absence or imperfection of *data* are no reasons for failing to make an explicit value judgement about the relative importance of mortality and morbidity. Finally, it assumes that all years of life lost are equal value regardless of whose life is involved and regardless of any discounting for the futurity of many of these life-years.

Chen (1973) made a number of changes to the formula in order to measure the differential ill health between a target and a reference population, eliminating D, introducing *relative* mortality and allowing for the fact that life expectancy in the absence of a specific disease is not likely to be the same for Indians and WASPS. His 'G index' was:

$$G = (M_i/M_a)(D_1 + D_2)$$

where M_i and M_a are as before, but unadjusted for age and sex, and

$D_1 = $ difference between observed and 'expected' years lost from disease-specific mortality in Indian population;

$D_2 = $ difference between observed and 'expected' years lost from disease-specific morbidity in Indian population. The 'expected' values were those that would obtain if the disease impact on Indian and US populations were the same.

Although the Chen G index has a different purpose from the Q index, the value assumptions it makes are, in fact, the same: the morbidity measures making up D_2 are weighted in the same 1:3 ratio and the mortality and morbidity elements are assigned equal weights of unity in terms of time. The G index measures the potential increase in health status from the complete elimination of a disease, while the Q index measures the increase if the target population is improved to the level of the reference population.

An alternative and perhaps more sympathetic interpretation would be to suppose that these weights are to be regarded as essentially *provisional*, to be altered in the light of professional (etc.) judgements about the validity of the index and after the experience of practical use. Indeed, both Miller and Chen argue strongly, and surely wisely, that such an index should not be used in isolation from or regardless of professional judgements. One might add that the judgements (of value) of politicians and patients who are important non-professionals should probably also have some role. As we shall see, other investigators have been far less leery about the explicit use of normative weights in index construction and have gone to quite sophisticated lengths to derive these.

It is also finally worth noting that both the Q and G indexes are not independent of inputs: an increase in hospital provision to the Indian relative to non-Indian population would increase both indexes, suggesting that 'need' has increased along with the means of meeting it. This is a highly undesirable feature of health indexes but is inherent in all measures based upon health care *processes*: increase the number of patients processed, and 'need' invariably rises.

There has of course been some debate as to whether it is really necessary to combine the dimensions into a single index, or at least into a set of indexes that is smaller than the total number of dimensions. In a very early study, for example, Stouman and Falk (1936) argued that a single combined index 'could have only a slight interest and might serve as much to obscure as to measure individuality of . . . problems'. While this point is well taken, there are clearly many occasions when it is desired to classify groups, regions and individuals according to their overall health status, to record changes in it over time and to relate changes in it to the various factors thought to influence it.

As we shall see, some thorny issues are raised once it is decided to combine different dimensions of ill health to make a single index; and, ultimately, there is no escaping the fact that at some stage in the decision-making hierarchy *someone* will have to apply *some* weights if any decision is to be reached. For example, someone will have to decide whether, in regional patterns of resource distribution, a region with high morbidity but lower mortality rates should receive more or less priority than one with high mortality but lower morbidity.

This problem cannot be escaped by disaggregation. For example, disaggregating mortality and morbidity according to the diseases associated with them will indicate the specific kind of resources required to combat them; but, so long as resources are not unlimited, it will not obviate the necessity of deciding which diseases are the more 'serious'. Precisely such an exercise, in which weights are assigned to diseases (but the weights are not variable with respect to prevalence or incidence), has been conducted for Ontario by Wolfson (1974). In cases, however, where a rather eclectic set of indicators is used to form merely impressionistic judgements of need, it would seem preferable not to combine them. Such applies, for example, when one uses existing data to make international comparisons. There is no obviously uniquely right way of adding up, say, crude mortality, perinatal mortality and maternal mortality rates in an international comparison study because the weights applicable in any one country, no matter how carefully they have been derived, may be quite inappropriate for another. This is merely one aspect of the familiar problem of interregional comparisons of standards of living.

There are two basic approaches to the question of weights once it has been decided that the dimensions measured are to be *thoughtfully* combined.

One, which we term the 'functional/dysfunctional' approach, ranks the dimensions by priority; for example, incontinence is a worse handicap than inability to work, which is, in turn, worse than being unable to go out shopping. The second, which we term the 'economic' approach, is more flexible allowing (i) that the degree of relative 'badness' of the above handicaps depends partly on their severity and (ii) that they may interact in such a way that a combination of disabilities may be worse (or better) than the sum of their 'badness' considered separately. The terms 'functional/dysfunctional' and 'economic' are used because the two approaches seem to be much in the spirit of the functionalist sociological and anthropological literature on the one hand and the economic theory of individual action on the other. Paradoxically, however, the functional/dysfunctional approach has been widely used by economists, medical researchers and operations researchers (as we have already seen in the Guttman scale), while sociologists have often been closer in their approach to the potential sensitivity of what we here describe as the 'economic' approach.

At least some economists have frowned on the first of these approaches (e.g. Olson, 1970; Culyer, 1973), partly because it can lead easily to logical error and triviality and partly, which is more relevant in the present context, because it consists of a highly unrealistic way of describing the kinds of values that people actually have; for example, it implies a 'lexicographic' preference ordering of the type that says all disability of the 'worst' category should be ameliorated before any of another category. Actually, it seems far more plausible to suppose that the ranking of categories of disability varies continuously according to the severity of disabilities in those categories, as postulated in Culyer, Lavers and Williams (1971).

If, then, a lexicographic approach seems too crude, at least at the level of abstraction needed for defining the *general* characteristics which a procedure for measuring health status ought to have, we must look more closely at the kind of 'measurement' that is implied by what we have called the 'economic' approach in contrast with the 'functional/dysfunctional' approach. Basically we shall be concerned with *ordinal* and *cardinal* measurement.

A purely ordinal scale of measurement gives only the rank order of entities. Once a number has been assigned to any one entity, the only constraint on the numbers assigned to the others is that successively higher entities have successively higher numbers and successively lower entities have successively lower ones. We may be concerned with two kinds of cardinal measurement. Measurement on an *interval* scale implies that numbers assigned to entities are arbitrary save that they not only order them (as in ordinal measurement) but also keep the ratio of the intervals between them the same. This kind of measure is akin to that which we use for measuring temperature: a temperature of 212°F may appear 'twice as hot' as 106°F; yet if we compared the same degrees of hotness on a Celsius scale, we could scarcely claim that

100°C were 'twice as hot', as 41.1°C. With interval scales, like measures of temperature, there is no special significance attached to zero, for the origin is arbitrary. But we can compare difference between temperature consistently. Thus the difference between 212°F and 106°F is twice that between 106°F and 53°F. Similarly, the difference between 100°C and 41.1°C is twice that between 41.1°C and 11.7°C. The second kind of cardinality, measurement on a *ratio* scale, does not have an arbitrary origin for the scale: for example, zero means 'none', and only the unit is arbitrary, so we can speak of 'twice as much' here as there, etc., as in measures of weight and measures of mortality, disease incidence, etc. This latter is the 'strongest' form of measurement we shall encounter.

Typically, in economics dimensions on axes are measured on a ratio scale (guns or butter) while value (utility) is measured either ordinally or on an interval scale. With health indexes, the axes may be ordinal (degrees of disability) or on a ratio scale (morbidity rates), while the values taken by the index combining the entities on the axes are typically on an interval scale.

The ways in which overall scores are assigned to various combinations of scores of the several dimensions that may be used are crucially determined by the kind of measurement being used. This we shall see as we examine some studies that have been undertaken. The nature of the measurement must also be borne in mind when interpreting the results, and here even the sophisticated have, as we shall see, been led astray.

One important and exceedingly thorough study (Harris *et al.*, 1971) sought to measure degrees of physical, mental and sensory handicap in the population in order to assess its effect on ability to obtain work, need for health and welfare support and so on. This study classified severity of handicap into eight categories varying from (i) 'people needing help going to or using the WC practically every night ... need to be fed and dressed or, if they can feed and/or dress themselves, they need a lot of help during the day with washing and WC, or are incontinent' to (viii) 'people to whom impairment presents no difficulty in taking care of themselves'. The first three of these categories, relating to those who need 'special care', were defined in terms of the presence or otherwise of specific inabilities or restrictions. The rest, however, were defined in terms of ratio scale scoring system for the degree of impairment or disability in specified dimensions subsequently combined to make only *ordinal* judgements, and is therefore of more interest in the present context. The dimensions, the units of measurement (verbal descriptions) and scores were as in table 2.3.

The procedure then was to add up the predetermined scores according to the technical assignment of individuals within the cells of table 2.3. The crucial value judgements relate, of course, (i) to the selection of the eight dimensions and (ii) to the relative (and fixed) weights assigned them. In fact, in this study degree of severity was not assessed by experts such as social workers but by the informants themselves: the experts provided the descrip-

TABLE 2.3

Dimensions, units of measurement and scores of the Harris index

Dimensions	Units of measurement of severity		
	Can do with no difficulty (a)	Some difficulty but can do on own (b)	Cannot do on own even with difficulty (c)
1 Getting in/ out of bed	0	2	3
2 Getting to/ using WC	0	4	6
3a Having bath	0	2	3
3b Washing hands and face	0	2	3
4 Putting on shoes/stockings	0	2	3
5 Doing up zips/ buttons	0	4	6
6 Dressing (other than 4 and 5)	0	2	3
7 Feeding	0	4	6
8 Combing or shaving	0	2	3

Source: Harris (1971, Appendix D).

tion of the units of measurement and the corresponding scores; respondents decided to which compartments they belonged.

If we take the simplification of the Harris approach used in an earlier discussion of its implications (Culyer, 1976, pp. 37ff.) we may construct figure 2.1. From the figure it may be seen that individuals may, on these two dimensions alone, fall into eight categories, with those who are least impaired receiving the index 0 and those most severely impaired receiving an index of 9. The interpretation of these numbers is ordinal – a score of 6 implying that a person is more handicapped than he would be with a score of 2 – but not ratio; viz. it is not intended to convey that he is three times worse off. The combination (b,b) (where the first letter refers to the ordinate, or vertical, axis) is, however, regarded as equally handicapping as the combination (a,c) (assuming, of course, no difference in any other dimensions not shown in the figure).

If combinations such as (b,b) are to remain 'equal to' combinations such as (a,c) it follows that, as we have pointed out above, the ordering of degrees of severity in each dimension has to be on a ratio scale, and that the ratio of increments in one dimension to those in any other remain constant. Thus, we could not merely double all the numbers assigned to difficulty in using the WC (0,4,6) and leave unchanged the numbers assigned to difficulty in getting out of bed. If we did (as the reader may readily compute for himself) combinations (b,b) and (a,c) would no longer be equivalent. If we double one lot we must therefore double the others. Nor could we take the order (0,4,5) as equivalent to (0,4,6) in the WC severity dimension, as we could if they were merely ordinal numbers, without having to change the numbers in the other dimension: in particular, to preserve the equality of (b,b) and (a,c), $b = 2$ have to become $b = 1$, while to keep $(c,b) < (b,c)$, $c < 2$ is required.

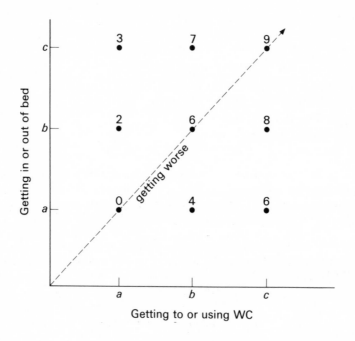

FIGURE 2.1

None of these implications were, of course, identified in the Harris study, and we should note that the apparent restrictiveness of an implicit ratio scale interpretation of the axes, and of their proportionality one to another, is much reduced by the merely ordinal interpretation of the resultant index of handicap. In general, however, it would seem undesirable to suppose that an index can be derived by simply adding up the scores on dimensions. In particular, if the total is no more than the sum of the parts, *no allowance is made for the possibility that one may wish to regard a combination of disabilities as worse than the sum of each considered separately.*

The way in which the index was used (i.e. to classify people into groups, having only an ordinal relationship one group with another) and its purposes (which did not include attempts to measure the effects of care on changing disability states or attempts to evaluate the 'worthwhileness' of such efforts), substantially reduces the significance of these criticisms, however, and it would plainly be unjust to criticise this study for lacking a sophistication it did not require. The study does serve, however, to bring out the richness – but also the practical complexity – of even a rather elementary method. Within this method, the Harris study displays highly commendable thoroughness and common sense.

2.2.3   Assigning index numbers to health states

In experimental work, five methods have been used to assign index numbers to health states. These procedures simultaneously combine the trading off of component dimensions and the assignment of overall scores. The methods are:

(i)   the 'category' method;
(ii)   the 'magnitude' method;
(iii) the 'equivalence' method;
(iv)   the 'standard gamble' method;
(v)   the 'time trade-off' method.

The first three of these have been used by Bush and his colleagues and we shall draw on their work in describing the procedures and their results. The other two have been used by several authors including Wolfson and Torrance. For these, we shall draw on their work.

The 'category' method. According to this method, individuals are given case descriptions and asked to ascribe numbers within a stated range such that equal differences in the numbers correspond to equal improvements or deteriorations in the overall health status ascribed to the subjects. Patrick, Bush and Chen (1973) used both graduate students in public administration and public health and professional members of the New York State Health Planning Commission and Advisory Council. The precise instructions given were:

Evaluate the desirability of each day by circling a number from 1 to 11 which shows how desirable each day seems to you. Each number represents an equal step on a scale of desirability such that 5 is one step more desirable than 4, 11 is one step more desirable than 10, and so forth. The label 'most desirable' is above category 11 and represents a day in the life of a person who was as healthy as possible on that day, i.e. performed his major and other activities, had no discernible symptoms, and walked and travelled about freely. The label 'least desirable' is below category 1 and represents a person who died during the day. All items fall between these two extremes, and you may use all 11 categories as you see fit. [Patrick *et al.*, 1973, p. 235]

Judges were not constrained to use integers. A feature of this method is that those assigning the numbers have to bear in mind that the same 'distance' between any two pairs of numbers on the index must in the judge's opinion represent the same improvement or deterioration in health status.

The 'magnitude' method. According to this method, the assigners are given case descriptions as before and asked to assign numbers within a stated range such that the ratio of any two numbers corresponds to the ratio of health states that the numbers measure. The instructions given by Patrick *et al.* in this case were as follows:

Evaluate the desirability of each day by writing in the score box a number which reflects how preferable each day seems to you. This standard item describes a day which has been given a score of 1000. It is a day in the life of a person who was as healthy as possible on that day. Every other day should be scored in relation to this standard description. For example, if the item seems half as desirable as the standard, then write in a score of 500. If the day appears a tenth as preferable as the standard, then write in a score of 100. You may use any whole number or fraction that is greater than zero and equal to or less than 1000. [Patrick *et al.*, 1973, p. 235]

By anchoring the magnitude scale at each end, clearly this method, as used by Patrick *et al.*, is conceptually equivalent to the category method, differing only in its experimental features and thus providing a test for the reliability of the category method. The conceptual equivalence of the two methods can be readily seen: if 4 is twice as good as 2 which is twice as good as 1, then the difference between 4 and 2 must be twice the difference between 2 and 1, so that each unit measures an equal 'amount' of good health.[6]

Torrance (1970, p. 99) proposed a 'direct measurement' technique in which the judge was asked first to rank all the described states including 'healthy' and 'dead'. He was then asked how many times worse he considered each relative to the one immediately higher in the preference ordering. States 'healthy' and 'dead' were given the values 1 and 0 respectively and the 'times worse' figures were used to compute the values for the other states. Because of the high abstraction involved with this method for the general practitioners used as his judges, however, the actual procedures used were the 'time trade-off' and 'standard gamble' approaches (see below).

The 'equivalence' method. According to this method, the assigners were given the same case descriptions as before and asked to assume that a unit of health is the same regardless of the person whom it describes. Subjects are then asked how many sick persons are equivalent in total health status to a given number of perfectly healthy persons. The precise instructions given by Patrick *et al.* were:

Suppose there are two groups of people, both of which will die immediately if not helped. You have the resources to keep one and only one of these groups alive for one more year, after which they will also die. The first group contains 100 people in a state of maximum health (standard). I want you to make a decision concerning the number of people in the second group. Persons in the second group are in a state of health lower than the standard [items in the booklet]. With each item in this booket, ask yourself this question: 'How many people in this state of health do I consider equivalent to the 100 people of the same age in the standard group?' Start with 100 and increase this number to the point at which you are not able to decide between the standard and comparison groups. You may use any number equal to or greater than 100. [Patrick et al., 1973, p. 236]

Letting I_h represent the index for a perfectly healthy person and I_s the index for a sick person, then with N_h representing the numbers of healthy persons and N_s the number of sick persons of a given type regarded as equivalent, the experiment asks the subjects to select N_s such that

$$I_h N_h = I_s N_s.$$

From this the ratios of the indexes can be readily obtained, viz:

$$I_s / I_h = N_h / N_s$$

and with one point on the scale fixed ($I_h = 1.0$) and N_h given ($= 100$), we have

$$I_s = 100 / N_s.$$

The 'standard gamble' method. This approach to deriving an index from descriptions of health states is based upon the utility theory sections of the classic by Von Neumann and Morgenstern (1953). It can be explained with the aid of figure 2.2. In this figure, the points A and B are located and ranked. Here we assume that B is judged to indicate worse health than A in the simple two-dimension world there depicted; thus if we are to derive an index of *ill* health, B will be assigned a higher number and is located on a higher index contour. The judges having valued A and B, we now assign arbitrary numbers to them. Letting $H(A)$ stand for the number assigned to A and as $H(H) > H(A)$) the ratio of the difference between $H(C)$ and $H(B)$, $H(B) = 2$. Now locate some other combination C such that $H(C) > H(A)$ and $H(C) > H(B)$. The standard gamble approach offers a way of assigning a number to C such that all three combinations (A, B and C) can be located on a linear scale: whatever the initial numbers assigned to A and B (so long as $H(B) = H(A)$) the ratio of the difference between $H(C)$ and $H(B)$, and $H(B)$ and $H(A)$ will be the same.

The procedure is as follows: confront the judge with a choice between (i) a gamble between C and A, such that he will get *either* C or A with some probability (but not both), and (ii) the certainty of B. The judge is then asked what probability (p) of getting C (or A) will make him indifferent between the gamble and the certainty. In effect, he is asked to choose a p such that:

$$H(B) = pH(A) + (1-p)H(C).$$

Clearly, from this equation, given values for $H(B)$, $H(A)$ and p, $H(C)$ is determined:

$$H(C) = \frac{H(B) - pH(A)}{1 - p}.$$

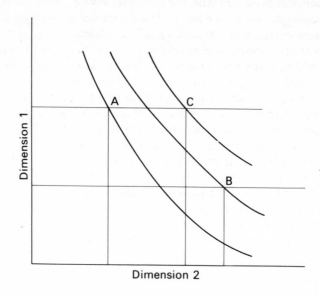

FIGURE 2.2

Suppose he becomes indifferent (the above equations hold) with $p = 0.6$. Then $H(C) = 3.5$. The judge, of course, need not be told any of the numbers initially assigned. He provides only the ordinal ranking and chooses the appropriate probability. To those who may doubt the uniqueness of this method of assigning numbers to health status (up to a linear transformation), table 2.4 provides some calculations given arbitrary numbers for $H(A)$ and $H(B)$, the judge's view that A is better than B is better than C and $p = 0.6$.

TABLE 2.4
The uniqueness of the standard gamble method of measurement

$H(A)$	$H(B)$	$H(C)$	$H(B)-H(A)$	$H(C)-H(B)$	$\dfrac{H(C)-H(B)}{H(B)-H(A)}$
1	2	3.5	1	1.5	1.5
1	4	8.5	3	4.5	1.5
3	6	10.5	3	4.5	1.5
6	100	241.0	94	141.0	1.5
100	101	102.5	1	1.5	1.5

The procedure can be applied to as many health states as one wishes without the necessity of comparing each of them directly with one another.

This procedure was used by Wolfson (1974) to rank the seriousness of ill health associated (by doctors) with a set of fifty-nine disease categories. Each physician was presented with the following option. Suppose he contracted a specified disease on the list: he had the choice of suffering it, with all its attendant consequences (including where relevant the possibility of death) and with its normal medical treatment, or of taking a hypothetical pill which would instantly remove the condition but had an attendant probability p of death. The probability was adjusted until indifference was obtained. Torrance (1970 and in subsequent studies) has proposed and used essentially similar techniques (and, indeed, pioneered them in the health field), with imaginative variations in experimental design in order to facilitate the judge's ability to respond in as ready a fashion as possible.

Although the standard gamble technique does not permit making statements like 'this state is twice as ill as that', (i.e. it does not provide a ratio scale), it does enable statements to be made about *changes* in health states of the sort: 'this change is twice as much as that change'. For most practical purposes, this is as much as is required.

The introduction of risk into the measurement procedure has both advantages and disadvantages. One advantage is that the procedure permits a method of combining indexes of components of the characteristics' bundle of 'health' into an overall index: the expected 'healthfulness' of two uncertain possibilities is simply their sum weighted by the probabilities of each component. This may prove to be of use in some applications. A possible disadvantage is that the health status index is itself not merely a function of the characteristics on the axes *but also of the judges' attitudes to risk*: a judge who was highly averse to risk, for example, would require a higher probability before he became indifferent between the sure thing and the gamble compared with a judge who enjoyed gambling. In situations where risk is inherent in the policy choice this is no disadvantage – indeed, it is an advantage. The standard gamble approach (though necessarily using physicians) is thus highly suited to epidemiological applications of health indexes, in prognosis, and in effectiveness studies where the outcome is uncertain. In descriptive studies, where the actual state of health is the focus rather than effecting some change in status, attitude to risk may distort the 'pure' trade-offs between dimensions of ill health.

This limitation of the standard gamble approach is inherent in Wolfson's study. Wolfson himself drew attention to the quite substantial coefficients of variation between probabilities selected by different judges (exceeding 50 per cent for twenty-seven out of fifty-nine disease categories) and, although he did not test to see whether some doctors were systematically more risk-averse than others, this (as well as the relatively small size of his sample) might have been a contributing factor to this large variability.

The 'time trade-off' method. Torrance (1970) pioneered this method, which is not dissimilar from the 'equivalence' method. Here, the judges (physicians) were asked first to rank in order of preference a set of health states. Let the states, after ranking, be numbered 1, 2, ... , n in descending order of preference. The judges were then asked what length of time x in the healthy state would be equivalent to the longer length of time t in a dysfunctional state, assuming death would immediately follow in each case. Assigning an index of 1 ($h_1 = 1$) to the most preferred state and $h_n = 0$ to death, the index for an intermediate state such as h_{n-1} could then be readily computed from the indifference equation

$$h_{n-1}t = h_1 x.$$

With $h_1 = 1$, it readily follows that

$$h_{n-1} = x/t.[7]$$

Torrance found a high correlation between the results of this method and the standard gamble, each of which gave internally consistent results, and concluded that they were equivalent methods. Both methods revealed, however, a substantial variation between the scores assigned to specific condition–treatment combinations by the eleven judges as Wolfson found in his application of the standard gamble. Torrance believed that the somewhat large confidence interval (at the 95 per cent level) would fall substantially for a larger sample than his eleven physicians.

In a subsequent experiment using larger samples of the public, Torrance (1976) found that, as between his time trade-off method, the standard gamble method and category scaling, the time trade-off method has the highest degree of reliability, closely followed by the standard gamble (which is, however, more complex to administer to the lay public). The category method was both less reliable and less valid than either of the former.[8] Again he found a substantial variation, however, in the seriousness with which the various disease states in this second experiment were regarded by respondents, partly perhaps owing to the judges' making their own further interpretation of the disabilities of each of the described states of health according to their knowledge, but partly no doubt owing to their different values.

2.3   A WAY FORWARD

It will be clear from our discussion that central issues of social philosophy and of health policy do not have to be left 'up in the air' at a level largely irrelevant for the actual operation of efficient and fair health services; indeed, they permeate all decisions and are, given specific content, intimately embodied in apparently quite technical issues – issues that, while technical, are emphatically not devoid of value judgement but are central to the idea of need advocated in this chapter.

Of the many implications to be drawn from the argument of the paper I would select two for particular prominence. The first concerns the training of personnel in the planning and management of health services, where it is important to ensure that the sophisticated practitioners of the more mathematical sciences in health planning (such as systems analysis and operations research) are aware of the values embodied in their procedures (which make them more than 'merely' scientific) and of the links that exist between these values (and the techniques in which they are embodied) and the ends of policy. It is also important, however, to ensure that the training of less numerate professionals includes a proper appreciation of the powerful potential of a marriage between systematic consideration of value in social philosophy and operational quantitative techniques for use in specific planning contexts.

The second important implication relates to the use of health status measures in policy-making. There is no question but that measures of health status are already used quite extensively within the NHS, though exactly how extensively is hard to say. Some are relatively informal and embodied in individual physicians' case notes. Others are similar to those discussed here and are used in the better research studies concerned with the effectiveness of treatments. Still others are macroscopic in nature, such as the use to which standardised mortality rates are put in regional resource allocation by the DHSS's Resource Allocation Working Party's report (DHSS, 1976). There is clearly a need for the extension of some of these techniques to be included in *all* micro-research studies into clinical effectiveness (see Cochrane, 1972; Rosser and Watts, 1972; Jennett, 1974; and Chapter 5, below) as well as their employment in more macro-decision-making, and more routine decision-making, to refine the current admittedly crude approximations of RAWP (Resource Allocation Working Party), or, at a less aggregate level, in drawing up district plans within the NHS to give meaningful content, which is capable of being monitored at regional level, to the 'GEN forms'.

Although it is not possible at this stage to specify a single 'best practice' independently of the purposes for which the need measures are to be used – their level of aggregation, etc. – there now exists sufficient experience with both the methodology and the practical problems of implementation, and the general rationale for such investigations is also sufficiently clear, for widespread experimentation with alternative techniques at many different levels within the NHS, in collaboration, where appropriate, with expert helpers from 'outside'. By the same token, an adequate conceptual foundation also exists for a nationwide periodic survey of health status in order to establish for the first time, independently of process and health delivery institutions, and in full cognisance of issues of both technique and value, the health needs and hence the health service (and other service) priorities of the nation.

NOTES

1. This paper draws on work by the author both published (Culyer, 1976) and unpublished

(Culyer, 1977). Its intellectual genealogy is traceable directly back to a joint paper (Culyer, Lavers and Williams, 1971). A discussion both wider ranging and more detailed is to be found in Culyer (1977).

2. Clearly (i) is really a logical corollary of (ii) but I prefer, for propaganda purposes, to leave the emphasis on prevention clear in the definition.

3. Other health needs not met as a result of meeting some specific health need are plainly costs in conventional economic usage. So are non-health needs that may go unmet. But so are other valued uses to which the resources may alternatively be put. Out of a range of feasible options, the most highly valued alternative use (which may not be in meeting a need in our sense) is the cost of meeting a need. It is not an immutable number and will depend upon institutional features of the relevant choice as well as the time-horizon, both of which affect the range of feasible alternatives.

4. Translation of the theoretical requirement that marginal impact on health status per pound be equalised for all client groups, regions, areas, etc. is, of course, easier to specify as a utopian ideal than as a practical rule of resource allocation. Nevertheless, practice should be informed by ideals, and progressively refined until an acceptable approximation is attained.

5. This is not a complete set of the value judgements involved. For example, we shall not discuss here the values implicit in trading off health gains with education gains; nor, at a much broader level, shall we discuss here the questions of value embodied in the general approach adopted in this paper with those, held by some to be different, embodied in a 'liberal' approach to health care allocation questions. Some of the former are discussed in Chapter 5 below, while the latter remain a fascinating prospect for future investigation.

6. A similar procedure has been used by Gustafson and Holloway (1975) to estimate the severity of burns: the severity of each dimension of a burn (e.g. site, thickness, area) was first scaled in this way. The scores were then weighted and summed. A study using a 'true' magnitude method is Wyler et al. (1968).

7. Although this method could be used for all intermediate states, a modified method was actually used for those intermediate states other than $n-1$ which avoided the continuous use of 'death' as a reference point. Judges were asked to consider what x would make them indifferent between h_{i+1} for time $t < x$ and the better (but not perfect) state h_i for time x, in each case assuming perfect health after the expiry of the relevant period. The relevant equality is then

$$h_r x = h_{i+1} t + h_1(x - t)$$

whence

$$h_i = 1 - \frac{t}{x}(1 - h_{i+1}).$$

8. Validity (the extent to which the index measures what it purports to measure) was tested by correlating the second two measures with the standard gamble index. Reliability (the extent to which the same subjects assign the same numbers to the same states a second time around) was tested by replicating questions in an ostensibly different form and also by a one-year follow-up test.

REFERENCES

Algie, J. (1972) 'Evaluation and Social Service Departments' in W. A. Laing (ed.) *Evaluation in the Health Services* pp. 13–18, London, Office of Health Economics.

Berg, R. L. (1973) *Health Status Indexes* Chicago, Hospital Research and Educational Trust.

Chen, M. K. (1973) 'The G Index for Program Priority' in Berg (1973).

Cochrane, A. L. (1972) *Effectiveness and Efficiency: Random Reflections on Health Services* London, Nuffield Provincial Hospitals Trust.

Culyer, A. J. (1973) '*Quids* without *Quos*: a Praxeological Approach' in A. Seldon (ed.) *The Economics of Charity* London, Institute of Economic Affairs.

Culyer, A. J. (1976) *Need and the National Health Service* London, Martin Robertson.

Culyer, A. J. (1977) 'Health Status Measures and Health Care Planning, with special reference to the province of Ontario' Toronto, Ontario Economic Council.

Culyer, A. J., Lavers, R. J. and Williams, Alan (1971) 'Social Indicators: Health' *Social Trends* no. 2.

Department of Health and Social Security (1976) *Sharing Resources for Health in England* London, HMSO.

Freidson, E. (1970) *Profession of Medicine: A Study of the Sociology of Applied Knowledge* New York, Dodd, Mead & Co.

Gustafson, D. H. and Holloway, D. C. (1975) 'A Decision Theory Approach to Measuring Severity in Illness' *Health Services Research* vol. 10.

Guttman, L. (1944) 'A Basis for Scaling Qualitative Data' *American Sociological Review* vol. 9.

Harris, A. *et al.* (1971) *Handicapped and Impaired in Great Britain* London, HMSO.

Jennett, B. (1974) 'Surgeon of the Seventies' *Journal of the Royal College of Surgeons of Edinburgh* vol. 19.

Katz. S., Ford, A. B., Maskowitz, R. W., Jackson, B. S. and Jaffe, M. W. (1963) 'The Index of ADL: a Standardized Measure of Biological and Psychosocial Function' *Journal of the American Medical Association* vol. 185.

Levine, D. S. and Yett, D. E. (1973) 'A Method for Constructing Proxy Measures of Health Status' in Berg (1973).

Miller, J. E. (1970) 'An Indicator to Aid Management in Assigning Program Priorities' *Public Health Reports* vol. 85.

Olson, M. (1970) 'An Analytic Framework for Social Reporting and Policy Analysis' *Annals of the American Academy of Political Science* March.

Patrick, D. L., Bush, J. W. and Chen, M. M. (1973) 'Methods of Measuring Levels of Well-Being for a Health Status Index' *Health Services Research* vol. 8.

Rosser, R. M. and Watts, V. C. (1972) 'The Measurement of Hospital Output' *International Journal of Epidemiology* vol. 1.

Skinner, D. E. and Yett, D. E. (1973) 'Debility Index for Long-Term Care Patients' in Berg (1973).

Stouman, K. and Falk, I. S. (1936) 'Health Indices: a Study of Objective Indices of Health in Relation to Environment and Sanitation' *League of Nations Quarterly Bulletin of the Health Organization* vol. 5.

Tenhouten, W. D. (1969) 'Scale Gradient Analysis: a Statistical Method for Constructing and Evaluating Guttman Scales' *Sociometry* vol. 32.

Torrance, G. W. (1970) *A Generalized Cost-Effectiveness Model for the Evaluation of Health Programs* Hamilton, McMaster University (Faculty of Business).

Torrance, G. W. (1976) 'Social Preferences for Health States: an Empirical Evaluation of Three Measurement Techniques' *Socioeconomic Planning Studies* vol. 10.

Turvey R. (1963) 'Present Value Versus Internal Rate of Return' *Economic Journal* vol. 73.

von Neumann, J. and Morgenstern, O. (1953) *The Theory of Games and Economic Behaviour* (3rd edn) New York, Wiley.

Wolfson, A. D. (1974) *A Health Index for Ontario* Toronto, Ministry of Treasury and Inter-governmental Affairs.

Wright, K. G. (1974) 'Alternative Measures of the Output of Social Programmes: the Elderly' in A. J. Culyer (ed.) *Economic Policies and Social Goals* pp. 239–72, London, Martin Robertson.

Wyler, A. R., Masuda, M. and Holmes, T. H. (1968) 'Seriousness of Illness Rating Scale' *Journal of Psychosomatic Research* vol. 11.

3. 'Need' – an Economic Exegesis

Alan Williams[1]

3.1 NEED AS A SUPPLY CONCEPT

A convenient starting point for an exegesis of the notion of 'need' is provided by the following quotation:[2]

The 'need' for medical care must be distinguished from the 'demand' for care and from the use of services or 'utilization'. A need for medical care exists when an individual has an illness or disability for which there is an effective and acceptable treatment or cure. It can be defined either in terms of the type of illness or disability causing the need or of the treatment or facilities for treatment required to meet it. A demand for care exists when an individual considers that he has a need and wishes to receive care. Utilization occurs when an individual actually receives care. Need is not necessarily expressed as demand, and demand is not necessarily followed by utilization, while, on the other hand, there can be demand and utilization without real underlying need for the particular service used. [Matthew, 1971, p. 27]

In this context 'need' is a quasi-supply concept: it means that a 'need' exists so long as the marginal productivity of some treatment input is positive. Only when the efficacy of treatment has become zero at the margin does 'need' disappear. People may still be sick, but since there is nothing we can do for them, the implication is that they are not in need.[3]

This interpretation also means that the last sentence in the quotation above could be rewritten so as to read: 'people may demand and utilise particular services even though the latter are totally ineffective.'[4] There are, of course, some difficult problems here concerning the content of the notion of 'effectiveness' as applied to medical services, which relate partly to physiological versus psychological aspects of medicine, and partly to the question, 'Who is the client?' A treatment, known to be ineffective in relation to the patient's physiological condition, may still be given as a demonstration (to him or his loved ones) that someone cares, and this may give satisfaction to them and indeed to other members of the community unknown to the patient who sympathise with the plight of the sick generally, so that the treatment may

32

be quite 'effective' in this broader sense. Strictly speaking, therefore, we would have to say that a treatment is ineffective only if it has none of the above good effects.[5]

Though seemingly odd in its implications, this usage of the term 'need' is common in political debate, which leads to a further important connotation, namely, that establishing 'need' is a factual, not an evaluative, matter. As one writer has said,

When we see statements to the effect that human beings need so many calories per day (and that states should make every effort to see that everyone gets this number) or that University teachers need books (which should therefore be allowed by the Inland Revenue as a claim for expenses) we may at first suppose that here is a justification for policies which ... appeals ... to an 'objective' or 'scientific' procedure by which 'needs' are established.

Whenever someone says 'X is needed' it always makes sense ... to ask what purpose it is needed for. Once an end is given it is indeed an 'objective' or 'scientific' matter to find out what conditions are necessary to bring it about.... The end in my first example might be mere survival, or good health, or the satisfaction of hunger; and differences in the 'needs' found by different studies might no doubt be attributed to differences in the end postulated.

When I say that 'need' is not by itself a justificatory principle, I mean that no statement to the effect that X is necessary in order to produce Y provides a reason for doing X. Before it can provide such a reason Y must be shown to be (or taken to be) a desirable end to pursue.... A *conclusive* reason would require showing that the cost of X (i.e. other desirable things which could be done instead of X) does not make it less advantageous than some alternative course of action. [Barry, 1965, pp. 47–8]

Thus the evaluative stage in the argument is pushed back one stage, but not avoided, and the statement 'X is needed' simply means 'X is conducive to the stated objective' or 'the marginal productivity of X is positive'. In order not to be pedantic in everyday discourse we may find that it is convenient to accept certain 'objectives' implicitly, and Barry sketches out the manner in which this is likely to manifest itself when we move from statements such as 'X is needed to produce Y' to statements such as 'A needs X', where A is a person:

At the core is physical health (e.g. the diet example); this extends more weakly to mental well-being (e.g. people need privacy, people need community). Then, spreading further out comes the performance of some function or the achievement of some object (the university lecturer example). Finally, we arrive at the fulfilment of some standard which can be independent of any function or purpose of the person to whom need is ascribed (old age pensioners need more money if their level of prosperity is to keep step with that of the rest of the community). The nearer to the core the use of 'need' is, the less linguistic propriety demands that the end be supplied in the sentence and, of course, the easier it is to suppose that a need can somehow be established independently of an end. [Barry, 1965, p. 49]

But it also carries with it the danger that the evaluative process is perverted so that analysts consciously strain at gnats while unconsciously swallowing camels!

3.2   NEED AS A DEMAND CONCEPT

We have so far interpreted 'need' to mean '*A* could benefit if he had *X*', i.e. *X* would be productive of something that is good for *A*. This confronts us with an issue that can no longer be shirked: '*Who* is to judge what is good for *A*?' or, in the terminology of need, 'Who assesses *A*'s needs?' We shall come later to the related question, '*How* are *A*'s needs to be assessed?'

A useful starting point is provided by the following schema,[6] in which three parties are distinguished, society (*S*), medical experts (*M*) and the individual (*I*), each party being asked two questions, namely:

(i)   Is the individual sick?
(ii) Is the individual in need of public care?

A third question is also asked, namely:
(iii) Does the individual demand public care?

But this is answered by observing 'those individuals who come in touch with the system of public care with a desire for consultation and treatment, and who are willing to wait if this cannot be provided at once' (Spek, 1972, p. 265). If 'yes' answers to (i) and (ii) are represented by *S*, *M*, *I* and 'no' answers by $\bar{S}$, $\bar{M}$ and $\bar{I}$ for each respective party, the outcomes could be represented as in figure 4.1 (Spek's figure 2, 1972, p. 266).

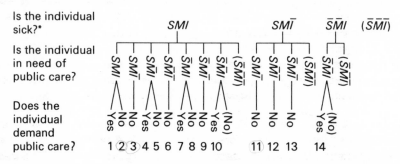

*The four cases $S\bar{M}I$, $S\bar{M}\bar{I}$, $\bar{S}MI$ and $\bar{S}M\bar{I}$ are disregarded in spite of their great interest. They must not be forgotten in a more detailed analysis. In addition we do not discuss differences in agreement among representatives of society and among medical experts.

FIGURE 3.1

Spek comments on this as follows:

Case 1 represents *justified* demand, with society and medical experts in agreement. Cases 2, 3, and 11 represent *latent need* with society and medical experts in agreement. Cases 5, 6, 7, 9, 12 and 13 represent latent need with society and medical experts in disagreement. Cases 10 and 14 represent unjustified demand with society and medical experts in agreement. Cases 4 and 7 represent demand with society and medical experts in disagreement.

...the answers to the first and second questions depend on knowledge and valuation, but they offer quite different educational and informational problems: this in turn will affect the ease with which the latent need in the different cases can be converted to demand, as well as unjustified demand suppressed. Latent need may also be defined as need together with absence of demand for public care. It is partly known through population studies and from individuals who, having contacted the system of public care, refuse to wait. This is not the place to discuss the problems which arise when society and medical experts are in disagreement on the latent need. If Case 4 is regarded as justified active demand, then it represents the thorny problem of how to have the doctors furnish the right care. If Case 7 is regarded as unjustified demand, it represents the thorny problem of 'over-use'. [Spek, 1972, pp. 265–7]

Bradshaw (1972) has a similar approach based on the presence or absence of the following four dichotomous discriminators:

(i)   normative need (i.e. 'that which the expert or professional, administrator or social scientist defines as need in any given situation. A "desirable" standard is laid down and is compared with the standard that actually exists');

(ii) felt need (i.e. 'Here need is equated with want. When assessing need for a service, the population is asked whether they feel they need it');

(iii) expressed need (i.e. 'Expressed need or demand is felt need turned into action.... Expressed need is commonly used in the health services where waiting-lists are taken as a measure of unmet need. Waiting-lists are generally accepted as a poor definition of "real need" – especially for pre-symptomatic cases');

(iv) comparative need (i.e. 'obtained by studying the characteristics of the population in receipt of a service. If there are people with similar characteristics not in receipt of a service, then they are in need').

The first thing to note is that the judgements of 'society' play no role in Bradshaw's taxonomy, only those of the individual and the experts. It will also be seen that Bradshaw's 'normative need' is equivalent to Spek's medical experts answering 'yes' to both questions (i) and (ii) (Spek's Cases 1, 2, 3, 7, 8, 9, 11 and 13). Bradshaw's 'felt need' is equivalent to Spek's *individual* answering 'yes' to those two questions (Spek's Cases 1, 2, 4, 5, 7, 8, 10 and 14). Bradshaw's 'expressed need' is equivalent to Spek's question (iii) being answered affirmatively (Spek's Cases 1, 4, 7, 10 and 14). Bradshaw's 'comparative need' seems to be approximately equivalent to Spek's 'latent need' (Cases 2, 3 and 11; but with 9 added since 'society's' adverse judgement is no longer relevant), where the individual does not demand the service even though the medical experts think he is sick and needs public care.

If we define 'need' as the situation in which the medical expert answers 'yes' to questions (i) and (ii), we could rewrite the original quotation from Matthew, expunging the words 'need' and 'demand', as follows:

The medical experts' judgement as to whether or not a person is sick and capable of benefiting from medical care must be distinguished from that person's use of services or 'utilisation'. A person is judged by medical experts to be capable of benefiting from medical care when that individual has an illness or disability for which they believe there is an effective and acceptable treatment or care. This phenomenon can be expressed either in terms of the type of illness or disability to which the treatment or care is directed, or in terms of the treatment or facilities for treatment themselves. An individual presents himself for treatment when he considers that he is sick and may be capable of benefiting from medical care, and wishes to avail himself of that possibility. Utilisation occurs when an individual actually receives care. An individual who would be judged by medical experts to be sick and capable of benefiting from medical care will not necessarily present himself and request treatment, and such requests are not necessarily complied with. On the other hand, there exist cases where individuals request treatment and get it even when medical experts (or society?) judge them not to be sick or not capable of benefiting from the particular service used.

So far so good, but we are still taking 'need' to be an on/off concept; i.e., we are interpreting it in an absolute rather than in a relative sense, and we need to move on to the language of 'priorities', already introduced tentatively and obliquely at the end of the first quotation from Barry above. Unfortunately this notion, which *prima facie* implies relative valuation, seems to be just as abused, and hence meaningless, as 'need' itself.

For instance, one eminent writer in this field (Butterfield, 1968) manages to include all the following statements in his argument for better management and more research in the British National Health Service:

Until there is some tangible prospect of our getting on top of the increasing demand by the public, often for conditions medical students despise, all imposed on limited medical personnel, there is scant possibility of securing the second prime priority, namely happy general practitioners and health workers. [p. 77]

Now the decision behind establishing priorities implies some objective.... Should one begin by asking, what are the urgent short-term priorities in medical care of the health service? ... Or would it be wiser to take a longer view, and to consider the ultimate medical Utopia as the challenge, and then examine the present situation and see how far it falls short and ask what one can do to move in the desired direction? ... [pp. 78–9]

The long term target must be perhaps an unattainable, but generally desirable, medical Utopia.... [p. 79]

The inauguration of the National Health Service changed the relationship between the medical profession and the public. Before, the Hippocratic Oath notwithstanding, doctors could and did take up a position (in certain cases) of being unable to do anything. With the coming of the National Health Service, I think we must make the assumption that the profession as a whole took the Hippocratic Oath with society as a whole and such evasion is becoming progressively less easy. If the patient is really dissatisifed, he widens his contacts with the National Health Service, re-duplicates his consultations in another hospital. He or she can demand and probably will get help somewhere in the end. It is not unreasonable therefore to rank the priorities in medicine in order of the distance from the symptoms, that is to say, first the patient, then his general practitioner, then the hospital and administrative organisations. [p. 82]

This eventually (Butterfield, 1968, pp. 191–2) leads to ten 'selected priorities', characterised respectively by the labels (1) 'the first priority...' (2) 'a very high priority' (3) 'urgently needed' (4) 'will have to be undertaken' (5) 'causing serious losses' (6) 'special attention must be given' (7) 'should be developed' (8) 'there is a good case for' (9) 'funds should be available for' (10) 'there seems a strong case for'.

It is obvious to an economist that what is missing here is the notion of 'trade-off' *at the margin* between one good thing and another. Listing items in an order of priority implies that, until the first is satisfied, you will not allocate resources to the second, and so on.[7] The oscillation, in the above quotation, between regarding the solution of short-term problems as a *precondition* for tackling long-term ones and fixing one's eyes on some unattainable Utopia and moving towards it willy nilly, is but a dramatic instance of this confused and unhelpful way of thinking. The question still remains, of course, as to *whose* judgements about these trade-offs we should accept, and Butterfield recognises clearly that society, the medical experts and individual patients all play a role here, and that their respective 'priorities' do not always coincide.

If we consider again the social context in which the term 'need' comes to be used by the protagonists in social debate, it is easy to see why someone like Marshall is led to conclude:

Needs, other than the basic needs of life and health, are subjective, that is, based on values. Economists can handle the concept of utility even though it is subjective because this concern is with conscious wants, or desires, which are expressed as demands....

Social policy's concept of need is based on a collective value system, working with a norm of need satisfaction which is collectively subjective, i.e. the norm reflects collectively acceptable views.

The aim of research and of social policy is to recognise this and to distinguish between unfelt needs, felt needs and conscious desires. [Marshall, 1973]

Considerations such as these led two of my colleagues and myself to conclude that:

the word 'need' ought to be banished from discussion of public policy, partly because of its ambiguity but also because ... the word is frequently used in ... 'arbitrary' senses.... Indeed ... in many public discussions it is difficult to tell, when someone says that 'society needs...' whether he means that *he* needs it, whether he means society ought to get it in *his* opinion, whether a *majority* of the members of society want it, or *all* of them want it. Nor is it clear whether it is 'needed' *regardless* of the cost to society. [Culyer, Lavers and Williams, 1972, p. 114]

But the literature of 'needology' does serve one useful purpose in alerting us to the complexity involved in expressing policy priorities in a key field of social policy such as health, where conflicting judgements are likely to be made by the various parties. Faced with this conflict, we should resist the temptation to allot any one party an overriding role by assigning to that party the sole right to use the prejudicial term 'need' with respect to its own judgements.

3.3   DEMAND AS A NEED CONCEPT

The time has at last come to permit the economists to occupy the centre of the stage, and I propose to do this by analysing their notion of 'demand' in terms of the 'need' categories we have been using hitherto.

In its simplest form this constitutes one individual's ordering of his own priorities as he sees them, this ordering being constrained by the resources at his command. In principle it does not take account of the judgements of 'society' or 'medical experts', except in so far as these have affected the individual's 'tastes', which are regarded as exogenous.[8] This simple view of demand therefore places it as equivalent to Bradshaw's 'expressed need' (and Spek's Cases 1, 4, 7, 10 and 14). The 'resources at the individual's command' usually means income, though it occasionally means wealth, or, exceptionally, information, skill, time, energy, etc. Thus in the ordinary discourse of economics the demand for medical care would be taken to mean the amount individuals are willing (and hence able) to pay for at some going price. It will be noted that this is the first time the notion of price has entered the discussion (though we did mention opportunity cost earlier), and it warrants further exploration.

In the context of the British National Health Service medical care can be taken, as a rough approximation, to be available at zero price, in the sense that patients pay virtually no fees. What the (potential) patient does have to be prepared to offer is time and energy (and he probably needs information about services and how to apply for them and skill in making his wishes known in some circumstances, too). To keep the argument as simple as possible, let us assume that it is only time that is required. It is this notion that underlies Bradshaw's notion of 'expressed need' and Spek's definition of demand as involving a willingness to wait. But this is itself ambiguous, since it fails to differentiate between two distinct situations, firstly, that where the individual is told to come back at some specified future time for treatment (e.g. being placed on a waiting list for a non-urgent operation) but is able to pursue his normal activities perfectly well in the meantime, and, secondly, that where the individual is kept waiting in circumstances (like a queue in a doctor's waiting room or where one is bedridden awaiting an operation) in which normal activities are severely disrupted during the waiting period. Only the latter can really constitute a time-price for medical care, which fits in with the usual 'demand' notions in economics.

Although there is no reason in principle to deny the legitimacy of this interpretation of 'demand', it does have significantly different implications from the 'usual' case. Firstly, the time-price that is 'paid' by the demander is not 'received' by the supplier, as it would be with a money price, so that the informational content of the 'offer' is less accessible to suppliers. Secondly, the distribution of time resources is different from the distribution of money resources, so that the pattern of demand that emerges has a different equity interpretation.[9] Thirdly, since the money value of time is likely to differ significantly from one person to another, a constant time-price implies inter-personal variations in money costs depending on the value of time.[10]

In what we have said so far, both the money price and the time-price elements (and the respective distributions of 'purchasing power' associated with them) have been interpreted in a strictly individualistic manner, in which each person is assumed to be not only the best but the sole judge of his own welfare. If we now extend the realm of discourse somewhat, we are led into rather deeper waters.[11] One generally acceptable extension involves paying explicit regard to any external effects generated by an individual's consumption of medical care. Thus we could think of *other* people having a 'demand' for some individual having (or *not* having!) medical care. The operational problems of giving effect to this 'demand' are considerable, however, and may lead us directly into the more contentious second extension of the argument, where 'society' judges whether an individual's own assess-ment of his own 'need' is to be accepted as it stands, augmented, diminished, or even rejected. This gets even more tricky when 'society' decides that the best people to act as a social filter to approve or reject individual demands are the medical experts! Hence our initially tidy 'demand' concept leads step by step back into the morass of needology from which many economists fondly imagine that they have escaped.

But it is possible to go still further in undermining the relevance of the classical demand function, by denying that people are the best judges of their own welfare, *even when externalities are absent*. This seems to me to be the essence of the discussion of merit goods, which rests on the assertion that someone else (society or the medical expert) is better able to judge what is in an individual's own interests than he is himself.[12] Economists are so steeped in 'consumer sovereignty' notions that there is enormously strong professional resistance to 'interfering' with people's preferences, even though such 'inter-ference' is a major avowed purpose of the educational system, commercial advertising and religious and cultural organisations. Moreover, even within these conditioning factors, the capacity for rational choice can legitimately be expected to diminish sharply when people are ill (and especially when they are psychologically disturbed), so that the marked resistance of econo-mists to the substitution of societal or 'expert' assessments for the individual's own assessments in this field seems to be based on rather weak ground. Why then should we so strongly resist Spek's 'latent need' and 'unjustified demand' concepts?

I turn finally to issues connected with the prevailing distribution of 'purchasing power', or, more generally, of 'access rights' to medical care. The use of the simplistic demand function, which operates only with money prices, implies acceptance of the existing distribution of money income (and wealth) as the ethically appropriate basis for determining the right to formulate 'requests' for access to medical care. It is, of course, possible to filter these requests by requiring that some forms of treatment can only be obtained on the authority of a medical expert,[13] hence the expression of 'demand' in this case is a necessary but not sufficient condition for treatment. But this does not of itself improve access for 'the poor'.

A zero money price with queuing generates a different set of 'demands' and implies that the distribution of time is a better ethical base on which to formulate requests for access. Again, a filtering process may be interposed, and British experience has led one well informed observer to conclude that, under such a system,

In practice the scope for an individual to regard himself as in 'want' of health care is virtually unlimited.... The factors which determine whether an individual consults a doctor or not are highly complex and far from fully understood.... There are also real costs involved in converting wants into demands. Deterrents include the necessary expenditure of time and energy plus, for example, such factors as concern not to overwork the doctor.... The knowledge that there are queues will obviously deter many would-be patients from demanding care. Indeed, in the long run demand will tend to gravitate towards whatever level of provision there happens to be.... Need is, in any case, a medical opinion not a medical fact.... Collectively the profession appears to reassess its conception of need in line with actual levels of provision ... What emerges as certain ... is that there will always be an excess demand for resources and a problem of rationing. In the market place this would be achieved by a price rise.... In the Health Service the problem of rationing has fallen to the medical and allied professions. Rationing, however, has never been explicitly organised but has hidden behind each doctor's clinical freedom to act solely in the interests of his patient. Any conflict of interest between patients has been implicitly resolved by the doctors' judgments as to their relative need for care and attention. The clinical freedom to differ widely as to their conception of need has led to inconsistencies of treatment between patients and to the allocation, without challenge, of scarce resources to medical practices of no proven value. [Cooper, 1974]

Thus changing the basis of formulating requests for access still leaves one facing the problem of assessing priorities ('relative needs').

There is a yet broader notion that could be adduced as a justification for 'need' as the central (though imperfect) concept in determining the pattern of medical care to be provided and its optimal distribution between individuals, namely that 'in communities and countries where egalitarian feeling is strong and a spirit of national sharing is general, a national health service may indeed be the most efficient means of satisfying these wants'.[14] Unfortunately, this generalised appeal to notions of social justice and social solidarity plunges us into still deeper water, where we have to consider the political processes by which 'communities and countries' articulate, disseminate and discriminate between rival views on such matters, and give them operational effect. It is not unlikely that this debate will be such that the *mode* of doing things becomes the central point, rather than what it is reasonable to expect will be achieved thereby, leading to that final reformulation in which someone asserts 'we *need* a National Health Service'. As I was saying at the beginning of Section 3.1...!

3.4   A RESOLUTION?

The conclusion I draw from all this is that, if economists insist on textbook notions of demand as the only proper way to go about assessing priorities in determining the amount and distribution of goods and services such as medical care, then they will miss important elements in the situation and (rightly) be discredited and disregarded by policy-makers. If through appeal to complex notions of externalities and merit goods they attempt to go beyond this simplistic interpretation of demand, they will be forced to unravel the same tangled skein of conflicting roles and judgements that the 'needologists' have been grappling with, and on which we economists have tended to pour scorn.

The heart of the matter, as I see it, is a societal judgement as to who shall play what role according to which rules. The parties in the 'who' bit are (i) patients and other potential beneficiaries, (ii) 'experts', (iii) politicians and (iv) the electorate at large. The roles to be played are 'advertisers', 'applicants', 'diagnosers', 'priority-setters', 'treatment-assigners' and 'researchers'. The rules consist of terms of reference and behavioural norms to guide choice within whatever area of discretion is so assigned.

There is neither time nor space here to do more than sketch out the lines along which an appropriate clarification and legitimation of roles within a medical care system might be developed, but in skeletal form it would be as follows.

(i)   The medical care system recognises that it has work to do *either* (a) because patients are brought to its notice 'spontaneously' *or* (b) because it has been agreed, as a matter of policy, to go out looking for them.

(ii)   Patients who are presented 'spontaneously' have to be assigned treatment modes (including 'no treatment') according to two distinct kinds of criteria: (a) whether they *could* benefit from treatment (a technical diagnostic judgement) and, if so, (b) whether it is worth while offering that treatment (a *social-valuation* judgement). Medical experts are clearly the appropriate people to play the former role, but are not so clearly entitled to play the latter role, unless society says so, and even then only within any 'guidelines' that society may lay down. This raises both (a) nice questions of principle about the limits of clinical freedom, the nature of professional ethics and the social, legal and moral sensibilities and responsibilities of medical experts, and (b) brutal practical problems concerning resource allocation, especially as regards investment (or non-investment) in facilities and skills that will enhance (or constrain) the capacity of medical experts to respond to the requests for treatment which are made to them.

(iii) The seeking of patients, via 'advertising' (i.e. information dissemination, 'education' and persuasion) or via more coercive measures (requiring vaccinations, certifying patients insane, etc.), raises all these same issues in still more acute form, and makes it still more important that one party does not usurp the legitimate role of another. Thus surveys of differential patterns of use, or of expenditure, or of the incidence of sickness, do not of themselves constitute conclusive evidence that 'something should be done', and proposals to conduct 'screening' tests to identify presymptomatic illness, even when curable, is to be subject to wider social valuation than medical expertise to determine whether any consequential treatment is of higher or lower priority than other uses of resources, and, indeed, whether the benefits of such campaigns are not outweighed by their 'costs' (in psychological as well as in material terms).[15]

(iv) There is clearly an important role for medical, psychological and sociological research in determining the 'technical' effectiveness of various modes of treatment (actual and potential), but again it needs to be stressed that to find a more 'effective' mode of treatment in this sense is not necessarily to recommend its adoption. It may be twice as effective as some existing mode, but four times as costly!

(v) Even if 'demand priorities' emanating in a simplistic way from 'the market' are rejected (or modified out of all recognition) as a basis for allocation of treatment, there may still be an important role for economists as 'technical experts' in estimating costs and benefits of other aspects of the situation, provided that the market can be taken as a good first approximation to society's valuations of these elements (such as the labour and material inputs of the medical care system, and loss of patients' and relatives' output from having people ill or under treatment). Again the well-recognised dangers exist of (a) failing to make clear the basis of valuation and illicitly supplying one's own values, (b) becoming so obsessed with GNP-oriented costs and benefits that others (pain, grief, suffering and loss of leisure) get neglected, and (c) overlooking distributional considerations.

(vi) The heaviest burden of responsibility falls on 'policy-makers', whose unenviable task it is to detect, clarify and give operational content to the 'wishes of society'. In this context the responsible policy-makers may be full-time 'politicians' (at national or local level) or citizens on a governing board, an advisory panel or a finance committee. The proper discharge of their responsibilities is made extremely difficult by the fact that many of the judgements they should make are usurped by others, and the information at their disposal is biased accordingly. They are the target of much of the confused and pejorative language of 'need', and are frequently poorly equipped to resist it in a constructively discriminating manner. They are thus encouraged (and often only too ready) to shuffle off their responsibilities to the 'experts', even though these 'experts' are *not* experts in the relevant matters.

My own conviction, therefore, is that we need to formalise these diverse elements in the medical care system in such a way that unambiguous communication between the respective parties becomes possible. This exegesis of 'need' is one small contribution to that task.[16]

NOTES

1. This paper was originally written for a conference organised by the International Seminar in Public Economics at Siena in September 1973 and was originally published in slightly different form in A. J. Culyer (ed.), *Economic Policies and Social Goals*, London, Martin Robertson, 1974. It reflects ideas generated in the course of work undertaken on the evaluation of public services financed by the Social Science Research Council (as part of the Public Sector Studies Programme at the Institute of Social and Economic Research in the University of York) and by the Department of Health and Social Security and the Institute of Municipal Treasurers and Accountants on output measurement in public services. I am grateful for comments and suggestions on an earlier draft received from Paul Burrows, Tony Culyer, Norman Glass, Alan Maynard, David Pole and Bernie Stafford.
2. Similar views are expressed in Office of Health Economics (1971).
3. There is a second stage interpretation of need which could be brought to bear here, which is epitomised in the statement, 'we need to find some way of curing cancer'. Here we are saying 'if only we had an effective treatment, people could be better off'. Since this raises the same issues of principle as arise at the first stage, it is not pursued further here.
4. A pungent polemic concerning the ineffectiveness of much medical care is provided by Cochrane (1972).
5. It will be obvious that because this notion of 'need' relates only to the *productivity* of the treatment (requiring it to be positive), it does not say anything about its 'cost-effectiveness'. Positive marginal productivity for a treatment is thus a necessary but not a sufficient condition for recommending its utilisation.
6. See Spek (1972). See also the discussions of 'need and demand' on pp. 315–17 of Hauser (1972).
7. Tribe (1972) also appears to take this view, in a peculiarly modified manner, in his section on 'lexical ordering', where he writes 'both individual and societal preference orderings might well display significant discontinuities ... without any strictly lexical principles ever operating'. Marshall concludes that all such preference statements are ultimately relativistic because

   needs are relative to the social situation, not merely to a particular type of civilisation or national culture, but to the differing circumstances of groups within such a civilisation or culture. It is also suggested that the system of values in relation to which needs are defined becomes incorporated into the individual personality. This means that the social environment influences, or even up to a point determines, not only what is felt as lack or deprivation, but also what is not felt as such by one group although it is by another. [Marshall, 1973]

8. This 'except...' may, however, provide loopholes large enough to drive the proverbial coach-and-horses through. For instance, individual preferences may be strongly influenced by medical 'advice', and/or by the prevailing state of public opinion concerning the 'rightness' of particular courses of action (e.g. abortion).
9. This is especially significant in systems that severely restrict the opportunities for substituting money prices for time-prices.
10. Smolensky, Tideman and Nichols observe that

    the good provided publicly at a congested facility is not a 'public good', but one whose implicit price is a function of the opportunity cost of time. A queue rations out users with a high opportunity cost of time, shifting them to quicker substitutes with a higher money cost. Instituting a money charge equal to the congestion costs of the marginal user will also ration customers out by the opportunity cost of time, but now it is those with high opportunity cost who will remain. In the absence of a social welfare function it is difficult to choose between these two devices. [1972, p. 101]

11. Charted more fully in Culyer (1971a).
12. An interesting recent examination of the implications of the Musgravian approach is to be found in Pazner (1972). Earlier explorations are to be found in Head (1966) and McLure (1968).
13. An interesting analysis of the implications of this sort of arrangement for the market for prescription-only drugs is contained in Liefmann-Keil (1974).
14. Lindsay (1973). But see also Culyer (1971b).
15. For instance, Thorner and Remein (1967) treat the exercise as a purely technical matter. A more circumspect view is expressed in Wilson and Jungner (1968), esp. pp. 26–39.
16. Some of the other elements are set out more fully in my recent paper (Williams, 1974).

REFERENCES

Barry, B. (1965) *Political Argument* London, Routledge and Kegan Paul.

Bradshaw, J. (1972) 'A Taxonomy of Social Need' in McLachlan (1972).

Butterfield, W. J. H. (1968) *Priorities in Medicine* London, Nuffield Provincial Hospitals Trust.

Canvin, R. W. and Pearson, N. G. (eds) (1973) *Needs of the Elderly*, University of Exeter.

Cochrane, A. L. (1972) *Effectiveness and Efficiency* London, Nuffield Provincial Hospitals Trust.

Cooper, M. H. (1974) 'The Economics of Need: The Experience of the British Health Service' in Perlman (1974).

Cooper, M. H. and Culyer, A. J. (eds) (1973) *Health Economics* Harmondsworth, Penguin.

Culyer, A. J. (1971a) 'The Nature of the Commodity "Health Care" and its Efficient Allocation', *Oxford Economic Papers* vol. 23 (2); reprinted as 'Is Medical Care Different?' in Cooper and Culyer (1973).

Culyer, A. J. (1971b) 'Medical Care and the Economics of Giving', *Economica* vol. XXXVIII, p. 151.

Culyer, A. J., Lavers, R. J. and Williams, Alan (1972) 'Health Indicators' in Shonfield and Shaw (1972).

Hauser, M. H. (ed.) (1972) *The Economics of Medical Care* London, Allen and Unwin.

Head, J. G. (1966) 'On Merit Goods', *Finanzarchiv* vol. 25.

Liefman-Keil, E. (1974) 'Consumer Protection, Incentives and Externalities in the Drug Market' in Perlman (1974).

Lindsay, C. M. (1973) 'Medical Care and Inequality' in Cooper and Culyer (1973).

McLachlan, G. (ed.) (1971) *Portfolio for Health* London, Oxford University Press.

McLachlan, G. (ed.) (1972) *Problems and Progress in Medical Care*, 7th series, London, Oxford University Press.

McLure, C. E. (1968) 'Merit Wants: a Normatively Empty Box', *Finanzarchiv* vol. 27.

Marshall, T. H. (1973) 'The Philosophy and History of Need' in Canvin and Pearson (1973).

Matthew, G. K. (1971) 'Measuring Need and Evaluating Services' in McLachlan (1971).

Mushkin, S. (ed.) (1972) *Public Prices for Public Products* Washington, DC, The Urban Institute.

Office of Health Economics (1971) *Prospects in Health*.

Pazner, E. A. (1972) 'Merit Wants and the Theory of Taxation' *Public Finance* vol. XXVII (4).

Perlman, Mark (ed.) (1974) *The Economics of Health and Medical Care*, Proceedings of a Conference Held by the International Economic Association at Tokyo, London, Macmillan.

Shonfield, A. and Shaw S. (eds) (1972) *Social Indicators and Social Policy* London, Heinemann.

Smolensky, E., Tideman, T. N. and Nichols, D. (1972) 'Waiting Time as a Congestion Charge' in Mushkin (1972).

Spek, J. E. (1972) 'On the Economic Analysis of Health and Medical Care in a Swedish Health District' in Hauser (1972).

Thorner, R. M. and Remein, Q. R. (1967) *Principles and Procedures in the Evaluation of Screening for Disease*, Public Health Monograph No. 67, Washington, DC, US Dept of HEW.

Tribe, L. (1972) 'Policy Science: Analysis or Ideology?', *Philosophy and Public Affairs.*

Williams, Aian (1974) 'Measuring the Effectiveness of Health Care Systems' in Perlman (1974).

Wilson, J. M. G. and Jungner, G. (1968) *Principles and Practice of Screening for Disease* WHO, Public Health Paper No. 34.

4. Output Measurement in Practice

K. G. Wright[1]

4.1 INTRODUCTION

Many people who are concerned with the administration of the health and personal social services see the advantages of developing output measures for the evaluation, planning and monitoring of their services. However, they frequently remark that output measurement is fine in theory but impossible in practice. My purpose here is to relate practice to theory in a chapter which should be seen as complementary to Chapter 2; to show that the development of output measures might be difficult but is not impossible. Although the example is taken from the services for the care of the elderly, the implications of the work for other health care policies are discussed where appropriate.

It may be as well to start with a cautionary note. The values that inevitably get built into an output measure are so important and prominent to those concerned with its development that it is easy to be hypnotised into a state of paralysis and to shy away completely from the task. The work described here was undertaken by Alan Williams and me at York University with considerable help on the data collection side from Jean Morton-Williams and her colleagues at Social and Community Planning Research. However, we were encouraged and helped by many people who are responsible for the overall administration and day-to-day delivery of the services for the care of the elderly in health and local authorities throughout the United Kingdom. As can be evidenced, we used their advice on many of the judgemental issues of value that Culyer analyses in Chapter 2 – on the definition of objectives, the dimensions of outputs, the components within each dimension and the weightings between these components. However, values did get built into the measure and the judgement involved is explained in the text.

4.2   THE DEVELOPMENT OF AN OUTPUT MEASURE FOR THE CARE OF THE ELDERLY

4.2.1   First steps

The output of public services is defined as their effectiveness in meeting their stated objectives. Thus the starting point of any exercise on output measurement in the public services is the definition of objectives. Usually it is very difficult to identify the objectives of public services, but we were fortunate enough to receive advice on objectives from many of the different professions (medical, nursing, social work, occupational therapy) concerned with providing services for the care of the elderly. These objectives were:

(i)   the maintenance of health and independence;
(ii)   social integration;
(iii) a satisfactory domiciliary and caring environment;
(iv)   the relief of the burden carried by families and friends in providing the long-term care of an old person.

This initial identification of objectives was reinforced by the eighth report of the Expenditure Committee (1972), which had received the following evidence on the objectives for the care of the elderly from officials of the Department of Health and Social Security:

General aims for the services can be formulated in terms such as 'to enable the elderly to maintain their independence and self-respect'; 'to enable them, so far as they are able and willing, to take part in and contribute to the normal range of social life of their community'; 'to enable them to live in their own homes as long as they wish and are reasonably able to do so'; 'to provide for essential needs which the elderly, with the help of their friends and families, cannot meet for themselves'; 'to provide treatment and care of an appropriate standard for those suffering from chronic disabilities'; 'to restore patients with illness or disability to as healthy a state as possible', etc. Even at this level of generality the possibility arises of conflicts between the ideals embodied in different aims. Thus a chronically sick old person may wish to stay in his own home though he could be looked after better (in a technical sense) and more economically in a residential home or hospital. It is necessary also to have regard to the welfare of the old person's family when setting aims and this can be in conflict with what is best for, or desired by, the old person himself.

This statement shows the complexity of policy objectives that occurs in most public services and is an early indication of the complexity of output measurement.[2] Some of the objectives are clearly in conflict, for example in finding the most appropriate place of care, or in the regard that has to be paid to the wishes of the old person relative to those of his principal helpers. Thus the development of the output measure faced two immediate problems: firstly, how to measure the achievement of any one of the set of objectives identified; secondly, if that is possible, how to combine these separate categories or dimensions of output into some general, overall measure of the effectiveness of policies for the care of the elderly.

The first task is difficult enough, but it is much easier than the second. Therefore, we decided to start work on one dimension to see how well we could progress on that before attempting any composite measure. It seemed to us more worth while to concentrate our efforts in this way than to dissipate them in making merely minor progress on all dimensions together.

After some preliminary discussions with our research consultative group and again with professional advisers, we decided to concentrate on the objective concerned with the maintenance of health and independence. This appeared to be an important, if not the most important, objective in the set identified. Moreover, there was a wealth of past studies which had attempted to measure dependency in an elderly population which served as a useful foundation on which to build. These studies had concentrated on estimating a person's ability to get around and to look after himself. Although they used different methods of measurement, there were common factors, and we decided to develop our measure from these. I have analysed these methods in another paper (Wright, 1974), so there is no need to go into the details here.

However, there was one important feature which does deserve some further consideration. This was the meaning of independence and dependency. There is a tendency in the policies for the care of the elderly to regard as independent only those people who stay in their own homes, and to regard the admission to residential home or hospital as a loss of that independence. However, we wished to free our measure of this idea, and to define independence as the ability to accomplish certain tasks without help from another person. Thus there is a spectrum of independence ranging from those who can carry out all the main tasks of daily living to those who are independent for very few of them or are completely dependent. This latter group of very dependent people may or may not be cared for in their own homes, and this definition of independence freed us from the false notion that all the independent people are cared for in their own homes and all the dependent people are cared for in residential homes and hospitals.

Related to this problem is the relationship between independence and health. One of the earliest criticisms we received of the measurement of independence was that it was too restricted and needed to include some consideration of mental state to bring it closer to a measure of the state of health. While good physical health is an important factor in the maintenance of independence, feelings of anxiety, depression and loneliness are important to health state but may not be reflected accurately in a person's abilities to carry out the activities of daily living.

Thus, it was thought that the development of an output measure for the maintenance of health and independence dimension should contain information about abilities to carry out the activities of daily living and about mental state. After a further period of intensive consultation, it was decided to develop an assessment schedule comprising three divisions, which were called mobility, capacity for self-care and mental state.

A four-part ranking was developed for each of these divisions, labelled 'high' (worst), 'medium', 'slight' and 'low'. The way in which the components of each of the divisions were grouped into the four rankings is set out in tables 4.1, 4.2 and 4.3.

TABLE 4.1
Mobility

Route no.	Questions Able to get in and out of bed and/or chair	Able to negotiate a level surface	Able to climb stairs	Able to go outdoors	Rank*	Comments
1	No	No	—	—	High	
2	No	Yes	No	No	High	Likely to apply to people able to propel a wheelchair
3	No	Yes	No	Yes	Medium	
4	Yes	No	—	—	High	
5	Yes	Yes	No	No	Medium	
6	Yes	Yes	No	Yes	Slight	
7	Yes	Yes	Yes	No	Medium	
8	Yes	Yes	Yes	Yes	Low	

The following combinations were not considered:

Yes	No	Yes	Yes	The inability to negotiate a level surface will make the last two questions redundant – see routes 4 and 1.
Yes	No	Yes	No	
Yes	No	No	Yes	
No	No	Yes	Yes	
No	No	No	Yes	
No	No	Yes	No	
No	Yes	Yes	No	See routes 2 and 3 – people using wheelchairs will be unable to climb stairs
No	Yes	Yes	Yes	

* High = most dependent.

These rankings were developed on the following principles. The ability to complete the task was recorded as negative if and only if a person needed help for that task from another person. Reliance on aids such as sticks, tripods, wheelchairs, handrails, etc. was counted as 'able'. Originally no distinction was made between the degrees of difficulty by which the task could be completed. This contrasted with a number of other studies which had attempted to measure independence using simple scoring systems. After

TABLE 4.2
Capacity for self-care

Route no.	Continent	Able to feed self	Able to wash self	Able to dress self	Able to make a hot drink	Able to cook a meal	Able to light fire*	Able to do essential shopping	Rank†
1	Yes	Yes	Yes	Yes	Yes	Yes	Yes	Yes	Low
2	Yes	Yes	Yes	Yes	Yes	Yes	Yes	No	Slight
3	Yes	Yes	Yes	Yes	Yes	Yes	No	Yes	Low
4	Yes	Yes	Yes	Yes	Yes	Yes	No	No	Slight
5	Yes	Yes	Yes	Yes	Yes	No	Yes	Yes	Slight
6	Yes	Yes	Yes	Yes	Yes	No	Yes	No	Slight
7	Yes	Yes	Yes	Yes	Yes	No	No	Yes	Slight
8	Yes	Yes	Yes	Yes	Yes	No	No	No	Medium
9	Yes	Yes	Yes	Yes	No	—	—	—	High
10	Yes	Yes	Yes	No	Yes	Yes	Yes	Yes	Low
11	Yes	Yes	Yes	No	Yes	Yes	Yes	No	Slight
12	Yes	Yes	Yes	No	Yes	Yes	No	No	Slight
13	Yes	Yes	Yes	No	Yes	Yes	No	No	Medium
14	Yes	Yes	Yes	No	Yes	No	Yes	Yes	Slight
15	Yes	Yes	Yes	No	Yes	No	Yes	No	Medium
16	Yes	Yes	Yes	No	Yes	No	No	—	Medium
17	Yes	Yes	Yes	No	No	—	—	—	High
18	Yes	Yes	No	Yes	Yes	Yes	Yes	Yes	Low
19	Yes	Yes	No	Yes	Yes	Yes	Yes	No	Slight
20	Yes	Yes	No	Yes	Yes	Yes	No	Yes	Slight
21	Yes	Yes	No	Yes	Yes	Yes	No	No	Medium
22	Yes	Yes	No	Yes	Yes	No	Yes	Yes	Slight
23	Yes	Yes	No	Yes	Yes	No	Yes	No	Medium
24	Yes	Yes	No	Yes	Yes	No	No	—	Medium
25	Yes	Yes	No	Yes	No	—	—	—	High
26	Yes	Yes	No	No	Yes	Yes	Yes	Yes	Slight
27	Yes	Yes	No	No	Yes	Yes	Yes	No	Medium
28	Yes	Yes	No	No	Yes	Yes	No	Yes	Medium
29	Yes	Yes	No	No	Yes	No	—	—	Medium
30	Yes	Yes	No	No	No	—	—	—	High
31	Yes	No	—	—	—	—	—	—	High
32	No	Yes	Yes	Yes	Yes	Yes	Yes	Yes	Low
33	No	Yes	Yes	Yes	Yes	Yes	Yes	No	Slight
34	No	Yes	Yes	Yes	Yes	Yes	No	Yes	Low
35	No	Yes	Yes	Yes	Yes	Yes	No	No	Slight
36	No	Yes	Yes	Yes	Yes	No	Yes	Yes	Slight
37	No	Yes	Yes	Yes	Yes	No	Yes	No	Slight
38	No	Yes	Yes	Yes	Yes	No	No	Yes	Slight
39	No	Yes	Yes	Yes	Yes	No	No	No	Medium
40	No	Yes	Yes	Yes	No	—	—	—	High
41	No	Yes	Yes	No	—	—	—	—	High
42	No	Yes	No	—	—	—	—	—	High
43	No	No	—	—	—	—	—	—	High

* Able to light a coal or gas fire or able to switch on an electric fire
† High = most dependent

TABLE 4.3
Mental state

HIGH	Severely confused – organic brain disease already diagnosed Often very depressed Often worried or upset without apparent reason
MEDIUM	Some evidence of confusion (e.g. occasional loss of memory, inability to organise shopping list) Quite depressed or often lonely Sometimes worried or upset without apparent reason
SLIGHT	Occasionally low in spirits or sometimes lonely Occasionally anxious
LOW	Little or no evidence of confusion, anxiety, depression or loneliness

some discussion it was decided to collect information on the difficulty of completing a task, since it cost little extra to include it in the questionnaire and we could compare the ordinal approach described above with a points scoring approach using the same data. This comparison is set out in Section 4.2.2.

A small-scale pilot survey was undertaken to test the scheme. Information on 360 people aged sixty-five and over was collected by some general practitioners and by the staff of the health and local authorities who had agreed to help us. The survey covered people in hospital, in local authority residential homes, in sheltered housing and in a variety of other accommodation in the community. This information proved to be of great help in sorting out many of the problems concerned with output measurement, as the following sections show.

4.2.2   *Different approaches to the development of the output measure*

A comparison between the ordinal system using the four-part ranking described and a simple scoring system is set out for the mobility division in tables 4.4 and 4.5.

Table 4.5 shows that there is very good correspondence between the two systems at both extremes; that is, where people can manage all the tasks or are unable to manage any. However, there is considerable overlap in the intermediate range from 10 to 20 points where one score often maps to three different orderings. This is to be expected on inspection of table 4.6 showing the possible range of scores for each ordering. There are two reasons why the orderings carry this overlap in scores. Firstly, the ordinal system

TABLE 4.4
Mobility

Abilities	Ease of completion	Score
1. Get into bed	Easily	1
2. Get out of bed	With a little difficulty	2
3. Sit down in a chair	With a lot of difficulty	3
4. Get up from a chair	Needs help or cannot do at all	4
5. Walk around the room		
6. Get up and down stairs		
7. Walk outdoors		
Scores range from 7 to 28	A further score of 2 was given to people who spent all their time confined to bed	

TABLE 4.5
Comparison of scores and order – mobility

Score	High	Medium	Slight	Low	Total
7	–	–	–	55	55
8	–	–	–	28	28
9	–	–	–	25	25
10	–	6	6	16	28
11	–	6	5	8	19
12	–	10	6	6	22
13	–	14	5	4	23
14	–	8	4	6	18
15	–	3	3	3	9
16	–	11	4	–	15
17	3	9	3	–	15
18	6	6	–	1	13
19	5	2	1	1	9
20	17	3	–	1	21
21	9	4	–	–	13
22	6	1	1	–	8
23	5	1	–	–	6
24	5	1	–	–	6
25	5	–	–	–	5
26	2	–	–	–	2
27	1	–	–	–	1
28	15	–	–	–	15
30	4	–	–	–	4
Total	83	85	38	154	360

ranks some categories higher than others. This can be seen where the ability to go outdoors is considered better than the ability to climb a small flight of stairs, since people who can do the former but not the latter are ranked 'slight' but those who can do the latter but not the former are ranked as 'medium'. In the scoring system the tasks carry equal weighting. Thus a person who could go outdoors but could not climb stairs would score the same number of points as one who could climb stairs but could not go outdoors provided that they could perform all the other tasks with equal facility.

TABLE 4.6
Relationship between the orderings and the possible range of scores

Mobility capability (from table 4.1)	Ordering	Possible range of scores (from table 4.4)
Bedfast, chairbound or unable to negotiate a level surface	High	16–30
Housebound (except for people able to go outdoors in self-propelled chairs)	Medium	10–26
Able to go outdoors but unable to climb a small flight of stairs	Slight	10–22
Able to manage all tasks	Low	7–21

The ordinal system has only four ranks and because of this certain achievements become irrelevant because of the inability to perform some other task. Thus the ability to get in or out of bed and the ability to get into or out of a chair count for nought if subsequently the person is unable to walk on a level surface, since all those who are unable to do this last task are ranked 'high' along with the bedfast and/or chairfast. Similarly, the ability to climb stairs is discounted in the ordering when people are housebound. On the other hand, the scoring system would allot four points separately to the inability to manage any of these tasks.

The second reason for the overlap is that the scoring system differentiates between four degrees of the ease of accomplishing the stated task whereas the ordinal system has the straight 'able'/'unable' dichotomy. Thus it is possible to pick up three points in each of the rated tasks and still be counted as 'able' under the ordinal system.

The score of twelve points usefully illustrates these points. It is shared by ten people rated 'medium', of which two are housebound and unable to climb a small flight of stairs and eight are housebound but are able to climb the stairs; by six people rated 'slight' who are not housebound but cannot climb stairs and by six people rated 'low' who can manage all the seven tasks but have some difficulty with between three and five of them.

The comparison of these two methods for the self-care and mental state divisions followed the same principles, so the full tables have not been produced here. In addition the self-care schedule was altered after a small pilot study of the questionnaire because the questions on making hot drinks and maintaining and lighting fires added little to the rankings, and, along with the questions on shopping and cooking, were applicable only to those being cared for in the community. Because of these problems, and because we wanted to use the measure to compare people being cared for in hospitals and local authority homes with those in the community, a restricted self-care division was developed using the abilities of washing, dressing, feeding and remaining continent which were comparable across all the situations.

Some information on self-care was retained because of its general importance. For example, the shopping question showed itself in some ways to be an important factor. In preliminary discussions our experts had told us that shopping was an important aspect of their assessment of the condition of an old person. If a person was able to complete the routine shopping, it was pretty certain he could manage with very little help from the statutory services. We found, however, it was difficult to use the 'shopping' information for ranking purposes because this ability depended not so much on personal capacity as on several general environmental problems such as the crossing of busy main roads, the distance from home to the shops and the need to climb steep gradients or steps on some part of the journey. Nevertheless, on a personal basis, if a person has been shopping regularly and is no longer able to do so, it is an important early warning sign to the social services that some form of domestic assistance is required.

Instead of repeating the comparisons between the two approaches for the other two divisions, it might be more interesting to use the two approaches to discuss the general problem of validity, sensitivity and reliability of measures.

The subject of validity is both complex and controversial in the social sciences because the constructs involved are frequently difficult to define. Basically, in searching for the validity of a measure one is asking whether it is actually measuring the property to be measured. As far as our output measure is concerned we are back to the objectives identified and asking whether the measure is recording the achievement of an objective. This is easier to answer in the case of dependency, because a person who cannot accomplish a certain task is clearly dependent on someone else to help. Generally, the ordered system is saying that the more people rely on others to accomplish a task, the more dependent they are. However, this is not true of the points-scoring system, which rates a person as generally worse off in some sense, the higher is the score of points. But this need not mean that he is more dependent, because people who can accomplish most tasks with some difficulty score higher points but are less dependent than some people who need help for some tasks but can do others with ease. The difficulties occur when one wishes to move from measuring the objective of maintaining independence to the objective concerned with the maintenance of health. In the first place the mobility and self-care divisions have to be augmented by the mental state division, and, while as we shall see later there is close correspondence between the self-care and mobility aspects, the mental state division had to be treated as a completely separate dimension, which then raises the problem of weighting between the divisions if a composite measure is to be obtained.

Secondly, although the dependency measure reflects the restriction of activity which is a common feature of the work on health status measurement, it omits another common feature, the degree of distress or painfulness experienced by the person. The work of Rosser and Watts (1974) has shown that it is possible for people to suffer little restriction of activity but a great deal of distress, and for others to suffer a large restriction in activity with little distress. These cases are represented in figure 4.1 below, where A is the point representing the case of little restriction in activity and a great deal of distress and B is the other case. There is no value-free way of stating whether point A represents a better health state than point B. People who particularly disliked inactivity and would be prepared to make great if painful efforts to overcome the restrictions would rank point A as preferable to point B, but people who found it hard to tolerate distress would probably prefer point B. Now, it might be argued that the points system is meeting some of these problems in its attempt to highlight the difficulties of completing tasks as well as counting the number of disabilities, while the unidimensional ordinal system is concerned only with estimations along the ordinate. In the ordinal system A is better than B because it represents less restriction in activity. However, the points system is trading off between A and B in a very simple and possibly misleading way, because it is quite easy for A and B to score the same points although many people would not consider them equivalent. It is the same problem that Culyer raises above over the scoring used in the survey of the handicapped and impaired (Harris *et al.*, 1971) and has generally worried us so much that we have tried hard to work with the ordinal system while recognising its limitations.

One of the problems we have faced with the ordinal method is that of sensitivity, that is, the capability of the measure to pick up changes in the property that is being measured. The sensitivity of the measures used is governed by the number of rankings included. Thus in the mobility division it can be seen that the ranking 'high' covers people who cannot get in or out of bed or in or out of a chair. Thus if the measure were used to track the progress of a patient and that patient's progress was such that after time he could get out of bed and sit on a chair for a while, but could not walk about, there would be no change in the ordering of his condition. He would

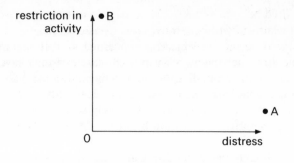

FIGURE 4.1

still be ranked as 'high'. If, however, we stretched the number of rankings to say, seven, then it would be possible to take such a change into account. We had a special reason for wanting a maximum of four ranks in each division,[3] but the general point here is that the sensitivity of the measure will depend on the number of items included, and the number of rankings into which they are to be ordered.

The degree of sensitivity required depends on the use to which the measure is to be put. If it is used for the routine daily assessment of a person's condition, it may well have to be very sensitive to pick up minor changes which can occur in such a short time. However, if one is concerned with only major changes over a long period of time the sensitivity can be reduced. Of course, the points-scoring system will be more sensitive than the ordinal system if it records the changes in the degrees of difficulty people experience in carrying out the tasks.

Increasing the sensitivity of a measure places heavy reliance on its reliability in the sense of both the accuracy and the dependability of the measure. The staff of Social and Community Planning Research carried out several tests on the reliability of the measure between different observers and found good results. There were some problems, especially in the mental state division, which would lead to some alterations in questions to be asked. The points system did bring problems because 'able with a little difficulty' and 'able with a lot of difficulty' were not easy to distinguish at times. A similar finding has occurred in measuring disability (Sainsbury, 1973), where a three-point scale ('no difficulty', 'some difficulty' and 'unable to do') was considered the most reliable that could then be achieved.

By this stage the balance of advantages lay with the ordinal scale. It involved less judgement and placed less strain on the reliability of the measure. However, it was concerned mainly with the assessment of independence and was far less sensitive than a scoring system would be. We consequently decided to see how far we could refine the ordinal approach to get over these disadvantages and the methods are described in the next section.

4.2.3   Simplifying the output measure

It was always difficult to work with three divisions in the output measure because of the problems of weighting between them. We therefore decided to see if it would be sensible to combine two of them by testing the relationships between them using linear correlations and principal components analysis.[4] The general correlations are set out in table 4.7. The mental state division was divided into three parts for the purpose of the analysis in order to test a larger number of relationships. The results of the principal components analysis gave very similar results with the mobility and self-care divisions grouping on the first component and the anxiety and depression parts grouping on the second.

TABLE 4.7
Correlation between the major divisions

Category	Mobility	Self-care	Anxiety	Depression
Self-care	0.70			
Anxiety	0.09*	0.15		
Depression	0.24	0.30	0.49	
Confusion	0.08*	0.00*	0.04*	0.06*

* Not statistically significant at 5 per cent level of confidence.

Of course, these results need interpreting with care since there are many different groups within this sample for which the relationships would not necessarily hold. For example, there is little correlation between the items in the confusion part of the questionnaire and the self-care facilities, but this is probably the result of having only a small (2 per cent) proportion of severely confused people in the sample. Other studies of senile dementia have found a close relationship between the severity of the dementia and the inability for personal care (Blessed *et al.*, 1968).

After careful consideration of these points, we felt that it would be justifiable to merge the mobility with the self-care division and to develop a revised ordering for measuring dependence. This is set out in table 4.8.

This new ordering closely followed the order set out by Katz *et al.* (1963), who found that in several illnesses people tended to lose functions in a given order and to regain them in the reverse order on recovery from illness. This is the same study that Culyer describes above in the Guttman scaling approach to the measurement of health status.

It is also interesting that the use of Guttman scaling to order disabilities followed a very similar ordering for Lambeth men and women in the community (Williams *et al.*, 1976), as shown in tables 4.9 and 4.10. This work means for the groups of people identified that it is possible, given the

TABLE 4.8

Mobility and self-care – a 'dependence' ordering

1. Rank all people able to go outdoors without help from another person (including washing and dressing)

	Mobility	Able to wash self	Able to dress self	Able to feed self	Continent
2.	Housebound	Yes	Yes	Yes	Yes
3.	Housebound	Yes	Yes	Yes	No
4.	Housebound	Yes	No	Yes	Yes
5.	Housebound	No	Yes	Yes	Yes
6.	Housebound	Yes	Yes	No	Yes
7.	Housebound	No	No	Yes	Yes
7.	Unable to get around the room	Yes	Yes	Yes	Yes
9.	Unable to get around the room	Yes	Yes	Yes	No
9.	Housebound	Yes	Yes	No	No
11.	Housebound	No	Yes	Yes	No
11.	Housebound	Yes	No	Yes	No
11.	Housebound	Yes	No	No	Yes
14.	Housebound	No	Yes	No	Yes
15.	Bedfast	Yes	No	Yes	Yes
15.	Unable to get around one room	Yes	No	Yes	Yes
17.	Unable to get around the room	No	Yes	Yes	Yes
18.	Housebound	No	No	Yes	No
18.	Unable to get around the room	Yes	Yes	No	Yes
20.	Housebound	No	No	No	Yes
20.	Unable to get around the room	No	No	Yes	Yes
22.	Unable to get around the room	Yes	Yes	No	No
23.	Unable to get around the room	No	Yes	Yes	No
23.	Unable to get around the room	Yes	No	Yes	No

TABLE 4.8—*cont.*

23. Unable to get around the room	Yes	No	No	Yes
23. Unable to get around the room	No	Yes	No	Yes
27. Bedfast	No	No	Yes	Yes
28. Bedfast	Yes	No	Yes	No
28. Bedfast	Yes	No	No	Yes
30. Housebound	Yes	No	No	No
31. Housebound	No	Yes	No	No
32. Unable to get around the room	No	No	Yes	No
33. Bedfast	No	No	Yes	No
34. Bedfast	Yes	No	No	No
34. Bedfast	No	No	No	Yes
34. Unable to get around the room	Yes	No	No	No
34. Unable to get around the room	No	Yes	No	No
34. Unable to get around the room	No	No	No	Yes
39. Housebound	No	No	No	No
39. Unable to get around the room	No	No	No	No
39. Bedfast	No	No	No	No

Comment: The general order of importance of functions is:

    (i)   feeding
    (ii) washing
    (iii) dressing
    (iv) continence

except where incontinence is accompanied by the inability to wash and/or dress.

number of disabilities suffered to say which ones they are, and to predict which is the next activity that the person will be unable to do. Thus, for the group of men in table 4.9, if it is known that they have four disabilities, it is reasonable to assume that they cannot dress without help and cannot manage any of the first three tasks concerned with mobility out of doors; and, although they can wash without help now, this is the next activity with which they will need help in the near future. Some preliminary analysis of our data indicates that we may well be able to replicate these scales for similar groups.

TABLE 4.9 Men		TABLE 4.10 Women	
No. of items disabled	Item disability added at each grade	No. of items disabled	Item disability added at each grade
1.	Cannot use bus or train unaccompanied	1.	Cannot do all own washing clothes, cleaning, shopping
2.	Does not use transport accompanied	2.	Does not use transport accompanied
3.	Does not walk out of doors unaccompanied	3.	Does not walk out of doors unaccompanied
4.	Cannot dress without help	4.	Cannot do all own cooking
5.	Cannot wash without help	5.	Cannot wash without help
6.	Cannot undress without help	6.	Cannot dress without help
7.	Cannot sit and stand without help	7.	Cannot undress without help
8.	Cannot use WC or commode without help	8.	Cannot use WC or commode without help
9.	Cannot get out of bed without help	9.	Cannot sit and stand without help
10.	Cannot eat without personal help	10.	Cannot get out of bed without help
		11.	Cannot eat without personal help

It is possible therefore to use ordinal measurement as a way of measuring dependency and disability and thereby to avoid many of the judgements that get built into the cardinal measures. However, the limitations of the method and the inevitability of judgement are plain when one reads the chapters by Culyer and Drummond (Chs 2 and 5). If we are to use these measures to improve the allocation of resources, then some relative valuation of the various dimensions of output has to be made to make it commensurable with the costs side. We are not yet in a position to develop these valuations, but we still feel that we could use the ordinal method to some advantage in the measurement of the effectiveness of the services.

4.3   THE USES OF OUTPUT MEASURES

It is easy to question the development of output measures. Why bother? Why take all this painstaking effort? The answers to these questions are in many of the chapters in this book. Output measures are essential to the efficient administration of the health and personal social services. They are needed for the evaluation and planning of the services; they are needed for the efficient allocation of resources; they are needed for making comparisons of the achievements of the health service in different parts of the country;

they are needed for comparisons of the performance of health services in different countries.

The work we did on the output of the services for the care of the elderly was originally designed for evaluative purposes. Evaluation of treatments in health care usually uses the well recognised framework of the random control trial so eloquently and forcefully advocated by Professor Cochrane (1972). In the care of the elderly it is very difficult to assign patients randomly to different places of treatment. Yet in a sense this is what occurs within the country as a whole, because people in very similar states of dependency are cared for in different ways in different parts of the country because of the local variations in the availability of resources. The provision of hospital beds, the places in local authority homes and the type and range of domiciliary services vary considerably throughout the country, and we sought to use this variation in an evaluative study which avoided the ethical problems that can occur in controlled trials.

The basic idea of the study was to draw a random sample of people receiving various forms of care in a locality for an initial assessment (e.g. all those in local authority residential homes; or 20 per cent of those being considered for home helps; or 10 per cent of those admitted to psychogeriatric units in hospitals; or 5 per cent of those presenting themselves at a GP's surgery). This stratification was to be left to local option, to be determined in the light of the anticipated workload that could be carried; but we were to be notified what the 'segment' was, and what randomising system was used to select respondents within it.

This initial assessment included information on the patient's dependency, mental state and background. The 'background information' comprised (i) some obvious social-economic data (age, sex, marital status, former occupation); (ii) a broad classification of any medical disorders (on a systemic basis, e.g. injuries or diseases of the skeletal system and skin; injuries or disease of the gastro-intestinal tract, etc.); (iii) a broad categorisation of physical environment (own home, local authority residential home, hospital ward, etc.) (iv) usage of medical and social support services (GP visits, home help, hospital outpatient visits, etc.); (v) social contact.

Three months after the first assessment a reassessment was to be made, bringing the background information up to date where necessary. This longitudinal approach, of reassessing the initial population at three-monthly intervals over a period of at least two years, was a distinctive feature of the research design. It was intended to produce data whose analytical potential increased throughout the period of the study.

It is obvious that the sampling procedure would preclude us from saying anything of general validity about 'the state of the elderly in Britain', because we would not have had a representative cross-section of the elderly in Britain, or even (except by chance) a representative cross-section of those coming into contact with the health and personal social services. However, our central interest lay in eliciting what factors in the background information 'explain' (in a statistical sense) *differences* in transitions from any given initial condition to the condition in which those people are observed 3, 6, 9 ... , 24 months later. Thus, if we found 500 people initially in some particular condition, it may be that three months later we find half of them still in that stage, but the other half scattered over five other conditions (one of which might be 'dead'). We would then try to discover whether, after standardising for age, medical condition and physical environment, the support services had any statistically significant effect on the probability of moving from one state to another.

The great problem with an exercise like this is to collect data on a large enough scale to ensure that there are sufficient observations in the number of transitions from one state to another to allow for the testing of hypotheses concerning the relationship between these transitions and the variables in the background information. The number of possible transitions is related to the sensitivity of the measure, since the greater the number of possible transitions, the greater the chance of picking up a change in the person's condition. The following examples illustrate the problems involved.

289 people were interviewed for one assessment and re-interviewed three months later where possible. The recorded change in condition as measured by two different schemes was as follows.

(i) Ordinal system (see table 4.8)

	Summary of Change	No.	Per cent
1.	Better	54	18.6
2.	Worse	41	14.2
3.	No change	158	54.9
4.	Died	26	9.0
5.	Ill or moved away	10	3.5
		289	

(ii) Points system

	Summary of Change	No.	Per cent
1.	Better	85	29.5
2.	Worse	99	34.4
3.	No change	69	23.9
4.	Died	26	9.0
5.	Ill or moved away	10	3.5
		289	

The more sensitive points system shows much more change than the ordinal system. However, the largest number of transitions from any one state to another was seven for the scoring system but twenty-two for the ordinal system. Consequently a much larger sample is required for the more sensitive system, and, of course, the cost of data collection will be so much higher.

The cost of data collection has hampered this experiment, and the feasibility of different methods had to be tested before we could undertake a longitudinal study of a sample of people receiving various forms of care as originally intended. However, it would be possible to use the ordinal measure to carry out a more restricted evaluation of, say, the effectiveness of various types of care for the elderly in local authority homes, without getting into the problems of a major data collection exercise.

The problems of data collection are usually greatest in an evaluative study because of the need to include information on all the factors that might affect changes in the client's condition. If one was concerned only with the assessment of the change in condition, the information can be collected in a very short time (two to three minutes). In fact, our schedules for ranking dependency and for mental state were designed to be kept as part of a patient's case record which would both help field workers, nurses and doctors to keep a check on the changes in condition and provide a useful data set for planning purposes. Such information would aid the discussion of appropriate methods of care because it would focus attention on the range of problems faced by a population, and on the type of personal help required to compensate for disability. There are often problems in deciding on the appropriate place of care that centre on the person's ability to look after himself and to cope with his environment, and the data on dependency and mental state, together with some of the background information such as age, medical condition, social contacts and environmental difficulties, would provide important criteria for aiding these decisions on a personal basis and for planning the development of resources for providing care.

Of course, this is not the only information that is required for planning purposes. There is an important need to cost the resources that are used to help people living in different places of care and to identify the most cost-effective forms of care. As stated in the discussion on objectives, there is a need for information on personal preferences for type of care and on the attitudes of the relatives and friends who often provide the main help to an old person in the community. Research into the problems of caring for the elderly and the information requirements of the joint care planning system in the health and personal social services will help to fill the gaps, as indeed we hope the development of our research will refine the work that has been done already.

Generally the struggle with the development of output measures has only just begun, but so far as we are concerned the work that has been completed, especially in the measurement of dependency, is an encouragement to continue. We have always recognised that progress along this road would be gradual rather than spectacular, and we hope that our optimism is shared by the many people who have helped us so much over the last few years. We shall, no doubt, be calling on their advice and co-operation again in the near future.

NOTES

1. Acknowledgement is made to the Chartered Institute of Public Finance and Accountancy and the Department of Health and Social Security for a grant to the Department of Economics and Related Studies and the Institute of Social and Economic Research at the University of York for research into output measurement for the public services.
2. It is, of course, debatable how far these objectives of the 'experts' coincide with those of the people receiving help, but a general debate on objectives has been avoided here in order to concentrate on measurement problems.
3. The reason was to keep down the sample size for the proposed longitudinal study as described in Section 4.3. Four rankings in three divisions meant that there were 64 ($= 4^3$) logically possible states in which to classify the sample; five rankings would have produced 125 states.
4. The detailed correlation matrix and latent vectors are omitted from this chapter, but can be obtained from the author.

REFERENCES

Blessed, G., Tomlinson, B. E. and Roth, M. (1968) 'The Association between Qualitative Measures of Dementia and Senile Change in the Cerebral Grey Matter of Elderly Subjects' *British Journal of Psychiatry*

Cochrane, A. L. (1972) *Effectiveness and Efficiency – Random Reflections on Health Services* London, Nuffield Provincial Hospitals Trust.

Expenditure Committee (1972) *Relationship of Expenditure to Needs* 8th Report, London, HMSO.

Harris, A. with Cox, E. and Smith, C. R. W. (1971) *Handicapped and Impaired in Great Britain* London, HMSO.

Katz, S., Ford, A. B., Moskowitz, R. W., Jackson, B. A. and Jaffe, M. W. (1963) 'Studies of Illness in the Aged – The Index of Independence in Activities of Daily Living' *Journal of the American Medical Association* vol. 185, pp. 914–19.

Rosser, R. and Watts, V. (1974) 'The Development of a Classification of Symptoms and Sickness and its Use to Measure the Output of a Hospital' in D. Lees and S. Shaw (eds), *Impairment, Disability and Handicap* London, Heinemann for the Social Science Research Council.

Sainsbury, S. (1973) *Measuring Disability* Occasional Papers in Social Administration No. 54 London, G. Bell and Sons Ltd.

Williams, R. G. A., Johnston, M., Willis, L. A. and Bennett, A. E. (1976) 'Disability: a Model and Measurement Technique' *British Journal of Preventive and Social Medicine* vol. 30, p. 71–8.

Wright, K. G. (1974) 'Alternative Measures of Output of Social Programmes: the Elderly' in A. J. Culyer (ed.), *Economic Policies and Social Goals* pp. 239–72, London, Martin Robertson.

PART II

Evaluating Services

5. Evaluation and the National Health Service

M. F. Drummond[1]

5.1 INTRODUCTION

For the purpose of this paper 'evaluation' is defined as the appraisal of alternative courses of action. This appraisal may be put in the form of two related questions:

(i) what should the objectives be?
(ii) are the chosen objectives being pursued in the 'best' possible way?

This distinction between objectives (ends) and the means of their fulfilment is largely one of convenience since many objectives themselves merely represent means to other ends. There may be a clear hierarchy of objectives; e.g., an objective such as the provision of a particular standard or type of service may itself be one way of achieving a 'higher level' objective such as bringing about an improvement in the health of a particular section of the community. Whether objectives fall into a clear hierarchy or not, alternatives will exist, both between ways of achieving given objectives and between the objectives themselves. Given the *scarcity* of resources, there is the necessity for choice; herein lies the scope for evaluation.[2]

Evaluation receives no special mention in the guidelines produced by the Royal Commission on the National Health Service (1976), but it is clearly pertinent to its task. Not least it is implicit in the terms of reference, 'To consider . . . the best use of the financial and manpower resources of the NHS'.

5.2 ECONOMICS AND EVALUATION IN THE NHS

The Commission itself points out that 'there is no universally acceptable set of simple criteria for deciding the best use of NHS resources' (Royal Commission, 1976). While this is acknowledged in principle (deciding upon what is best unavoidably involves value judgements), it will be argued that the criterion of *economic efficiency* is an important criterion to be applied in

67

Could use instead of allocative & technical efficiency but in introduction.

deciding upon what is the best use of resources. The overall objective implied by the adoption of efficiency as the criterion in evaluation is that of using available resources so as to generate the largest possible social benefit. In the appraisal of alternatives in health care, this will imply the selection of those treatments or procedures that generate the largest excess of social benefit (gain to the community) over social cost (the sacrifice made by the community). Sacrifices are always necessary when engaging in health treatments, since all treatments consume scarce resources. In consuming resources, the community forgoes the benefits that these would have produced if used in another activity.

It is a feature of economic evaluation that it considers the value both of the inputs (resources) used and of the outputs produced by the courses of action being appraised.[3] This is not true of all evaluative frameworks. For instance, medical evaluation considers only the effectiveness of treatments, not the value of the resources that these consume. Other procedures, such as the comparison of unit expenditures between institutions, amount to a monitoring of inputs without regard for the effect or output that those inputs produce. (Such alternative evaluative frameworks are discussed in Sections 5.4.1 and 5.4.2 below.)

Another feature of economic evaluation is that (in theory at least) the community is viewed as a collection of individuals, and that it is those individuals' valuations (of the costs that they incur and of the benefits that they receive) that are the relevant ones.[4] This is particularly pertinent bearing in mind the Royal Commission's view that 'the NHS should be responsive to the public's wishes' (Royal Commission, 1976).

The advocacy of economic efficiency as a criterion for choice between alternatives in health care implies the following.

(i) The efficiency criterion considers that gains (benefits) and losses (costs) in *all* sections of the community are relevant. Therefore, it will be erroneous (in economic terms) to consider the 'best use of *NHS* resources' without also considering the wider effects of NHS resource-utilisation.

For example, the trend towards early discharge from hospital, and towards more care in the home, may reduce NHS resource-utilisation (per inpatient case or in total). However, this reduction may be partly offset by (say) the removal of a relative from the workforce in order to care for the patient, and increased consumption of both local authority and the patient's own resources (e.g. heating a home that may otherwise remain unheated). The commitment of NHS resources always necessitates the commitment of other community resources. If a patient is to be treated, he must present himself for treatment, thereby at least committing his time.

(ii) In its usual form, economic evaluation is indifferent to which members of the community bear costs or receive benefits. Rather, it is interested in the costs and benefits generated in the community as a whole. The normal (explicit or implicit) assumption is that, if gainers from a particular course of action *could* compensate the losers (irrespective of whether they actually *do* compensate them), then that course of action is, on balance, socially beneficial. While acknowledging that economics traditionally does not deal with such distributional effects (other than to point them out), it must be said that it is often difficult to decide what is 'desirable' or 'best' in these matters.

For instance, suppose that, in the example given above, the early discharge policy is found to be less costly to the community as a whole. However, under the early discharge policy the patient may be bearing a greater proportion of the cost of his illness. It may be that in this case the amounts are small, and also the patient may prefer to be at home. Therefore the choice of treatment mode is not one of great *distributional* consequence. Nevertheless, a decision (say) to expand domiciliary care for the elderly may impose on the families of clients a much higher cost even though the cost to the community *as a whole* may be lower than for institutional care. The issue becomes even more complicated if (as is likely) clients themselves are not indifferent between domiciliary and institutional care. Economic analysts usually confine themselves to pointing such effects out. In any case it is argued that such effects can be nullified by compensation arrangements[5] and should therefore be treated separately from efficiency considerations.

(iii) In advocating the efficiency criterion one does not deny that objectives other than the maximisation of social benefit may be pursued. One such objective may be that of equal availability of health care for all groups in the community. The 1946 NHS Bill aimed to create a system of health services 'available to everyone regardless of financial means, age, sex, employment or vocation, area of residence or insurance qualification'.

The existence of other objectives need not imply the abandonment of the efficiency criterion, although the evaluation performed may be more restricted. In the case of equal availability, for instance, it would be possible to decide arbitrarily the shares of total health resources to be allocated to particular groups in the community. Then one could evaluate alternative procedures to determine the most efficient way of caring for each group. (The procedure of setting out broad guidelines for resource allocation between different care groups seems to have been followed by DHSS (1976a) in a recent consultative document.)

(iv) In promoting economic evaluation the importance of other evaluative frameworks is not denied. Of course, economic evaluation will depend to a large extent upon *technical* evaluation of health care alternatives for the estimation of key parameters. For instance, much economic evaluation will require estimation of the medical effectiveness of health treatments. Therefore, the advocacy of economic evaluation will imply the encouragement of medical evaluation also, although there are limitations of the use of medical evaluation alone. These are explained in Section 5.4.2.

5.3   STATE OF THE ART IN ECONOMIC EVALUATION IN HEALTH CARE

5.3.1   A classification of cost–benefit studies

The practice of economic evaluation in health care is to be found in studies of the cost–benefit and cost effectiveness type. Here, health treatment alternatives are evaluated through consideration of the costs and benefits that they generate. Costs and benefits to *all* members of the community are (in theory) considered, and total (social) benefit is compared with total (social) cost. In a full cost–benefit study, costs and benefits are made commensurate with one another through the use of a common *numeraire* (usually money), whereas in a cost effectiveness study benefits may be quantified in physical units (such as years of life gained) rather than in money terms. The choice of approach depends primarily on the question being asked. If the objectives themselves are not being questioned (i.e. if it has already been decided to employ health treatments to ameliorate a particular condition), then cost effectiveness analysis may sometimes (but not always) suffice. In other instances, particularly if one wishes to choose between objectives (e.g. the amelioration of one condition as opposed to another), cost–benefit analysis will be necessary. Often the analyst's choice of approach may also be influenced by practical difficulties, particularly where the benefits of treatments are difficult to express in money terms. Therefore, although the intention may be to choose between objectives, a cost effectiveness study (or incomplete cost–benefit study) may be undertaken to provide the decision-maker with more information, even though the final decision will require him to place his own values (either explicitly or implicitly) on benefits.

Several studies of the cost–benefit and cost effectiveness type have been reviewed by Williams (1974). In particular he identifies the types of decision that such studies have been (or could be) applied to. For example, the study by Wager (1972) considered *alternative places of treatment* (institutional versus domiciliary care) for the elderly. Alternatively, the study by Pole (1971) considered *alternative times of treatment* (prevention through early detection or cure at the symptomatic stage) for pulmonary tuberculosis. Other decisions to which studies may be relevant include choices between *alternative types of treatment* for a particular group of patients, or between *alternative client groups* (e.g. the provision of care for the elderly or the mentally handicapped), the latter being a particularly difficult choice.

However, such studies vary greatly both in their range of coverage (from cost-only or benefit-only studies, to full cost–benefit studies) and in their level of sophistication (from 'back-of-the-envelope' studies to those allied to a full prospective clinical trial). Over fifty studies have now been classified (Drummond, 1976) in order to illustrate these differences in approach. Many attributes of the studies have been examined and those itemised here seem to highlight some of the main evaluative issues.

(a) What (evaluative) question does the study attempt to answer?

Examples of questions to which studies have addressed themselves are:

(i)   What is the cost of treatment?
(ii) What is (or would be) the benefit from treatment?
(iii) What is the most economical way to treat a particular condition?
(iv) Is treatment worthwhile? (i.e., is it to be preferred to 'doing nothing' or to performing other treatments?)

Questions (i) and (ii) consider only half of the full evaluation problem. That is, they may consider outputs but not inputs, or vice versa. However, it can be seen that questions (iii) and (iv) are equivalent to the evaluative questions set out in Section 5.1 above.

(b) What range of costs and benefits does the study consider?

The relevant costs and benefits resulting from the employment of health treatments will be those relating to:

(i)   changes in health service resources;
(ii) changes in other community resources
        e.g. resources of other public bodies (e.g. local authorities); voluntary resources; patient's resources;
(iii) changes in productive output;
(iv) changes in health state *per se*.

For a full economic evaluation, costs and benefits relating to *all* of these must be included. In the past studies have placed much emphasis on changes (i) and (iii), suggesting (quite erroneously) that economic evaluation is synonymous with examination of merely the financial aspects of health treatments. Changes in health state *per se* have tended to be omitted mainly because of the difficulties in their quantification and valuation in money terms. However, there are some signs that this may be changing (Chapter 2 above). There appears to be less excuse for the omission of changes in other community resources. For example, information on expenditure of patients' personal time and money in obtaining treatment is difficult but not impossible to obtain.

(c) To what extent have costs and benefits been valued, and by what method?

One can view the valuation process as consisting of three stages, enumeration, quantification (in physical units) and explicit valuation (in money terms).

All three stages are important. The importance of enumeration is increased when, owing to practical difficulties, only some of the relevant costs and benefits can be quantified and valued. Then the decision-maker may have to make his own judgement of the unmeasured as against the measured. At the quantification stage the economic analyst will often rely heavily on parameters, such as the effectiveness of medical treatments, estimated through medical research. It should be noted that quantification itself is not value-free. The quantification of health improvement (for instance) requires judgements about the choice of the dimensions of measurement of such improvement and the method of measurement.

The most important aspect of the method of explicit valuation is the *source* of values. A number of sources have been used.

(i) *Market values.* Where markets exist for the inputs used by, or for the outputs produced by, health treatments, it is common practice to use existing market prices as a basis for valuation. Often these prices are used without adjustment; e.g. one estimate of the cost of labour inputs to a health treatment could be based on the salaries (i.e. market wage rates) paid to staff involved in that treatment.

Occasionally the existing prices are adjusted before inclusion in the analysis. Adjustments are made when the analyst has reason to believe that prices are 'artificially' high or low through the existence of a tax or a subsidy, or of market imperfections such as monopoly power. An example of an adjustment would be that made by Wager (1972), who deducted taxes on transport (motor fuel duty, motor vehicle duty and purchase tax on vehicles) in his estimation of the costs of home nursing.

Another market-based approach to valuation is used when, although a good or service is (implicitly) traded against others, the market does not generate a price (or set of prices) for the good in question. An example here is in the valuation of the patient's personal time. That is, time spent in travelling to or from health facilities, in waiting for treatment, or in undergoing treatment. Time is sometimes valued by *imputing* a value based on observation of individuals' behaviour in a situation where time savings are traded-off against extra money outlays.

(ii) *Policy-makers' values.* These can be elicited from actual policy decisions. For example, the cost of implementing safety legislation can be used to derive an (implicit) estimate of the value of life, although in most cases safety measures reduce the risk of permanent or temporary disability as well as of death.

(iii) *Professional judgement.* The values of health professionals have been used by Bush *et al.* (1973) and Torrance *et al.* (1973) in deriving relative (non-money) valuations of the desirability of particular health states. Another professional judgement used is that made by judges in awarding compensation (for loss of life or permanent disability) to victims or their relatives. Rosser and Watts (1972) have used court awards to obtain relative valuations of the desirability of particular health states.

᛭ (iv) *Clients' values.* These are likely to be increasingly used for valuing the desirability of one health state against another, although few examples exist at the moment. One example is the work of Jones-Lee (1976), who obtained estimates from individuals of the value of their own lives by presenting them (through a questionnaire) with a hypothetical situation where safety (reduction in the risk of death) is to be traded off against money outlays.

Each of the methods of valuation identified here has its own rationale, and each of them necessitates the adoption of a particular set of value judgements. For instance, the use of (say) professional judgement as a source of values violates the principle that individuals are the best judges of their own welfare. On the other hand, market values derive from the prevailing distribution of income, and therefore their adoption implies, in the absence of adjustment, acceptance of the prevailing income distribution. Whatever the source of valuation, studies of the cost–benefit type have the advantage that the method of valuation is made explicit. This is to be preferred to approaches that leave the (unavoidable) process of valuation obscure, since it enables reasons for disagreement with the implications to be identified explicitly and changes made, if deemed appropriate.

5.3.2   Observations on current practice

Further to the review and classification of studies, the following observations can be made.

(i) Progress (from *circa* 1960 to the present day) has been such that it is possible to distil a 'best practice' from the body of studies which, if applied *in toto* in a single study, would be likely to bring about an improvement in approach.

(ii) Many technical problems still exist, particularly in the difficult area of valuation of changes in health state. However, some of the work already cited suggests that progress is being made even in this area. Jones-Lee (1976) and Acton (1973, 1975) obtained *direct* estimates from individuals of the value in money terms of changes in their own health state and that of others. Another approach being pursued is that of *relative* (viz. non-money) valuation of health states. The best-known British work is that of Rosser and Watts (1972, 1974), where relative valuations of 'distress-disability' states are obtained by reference to court awards. In North America Bush *et al.* (1973) have derived a three-dimensional index of health states for use in evaluating a PKU screening programme, and Torrance *et al.* (1973) have used a similar index in the evaluation of a number of health programmes (e.g. a screening programme for the prevention of haemolytic disease of the newborn, a tuberculosis screening programme and a kidney dialysis and transplantation programme).

While no one would deny the need for more validation of such output measures, the work so far has shown that it is possible to approach these issues in a formal way. (After all, many of these issues are being faced by clinicians, albeit informally, all the time.) Also, the work so far has highlighted several important issues inherent in output measurement that previously were afforded little discussion. (For a fuller discussion of the principles and practice of output measurement see Chapters 2 and 4 above.)

(iii) The difficulties inherent in output measurement can sometimes be avoided, provided that one is content merely to appraise two ways of meeting the same treatment objective, rather than to question the objectives themselves. Two methods of simplification exist.

(a) *Selection of two alternatives for which the changes in health state observed are equivalent.* For instance, Piachaud and Weddell (1972) compared the costs of injection-compression sclerotherapy and surgery alternatives for the treatment of varicose veins. The medical outcomes of the two treatments, assessed through a randomised–controlled clinical trial with three-year follow-up, were found to be equivalent.

A further example is the comparison of day surgery and traditional inpatient confinement for hernia repair (Russell *et al.*, 1977).

(b) *Comparison of treatments where a single, easily measurable, component of output is paramount.* An example here is the case of chronic renal failure, where the patient (who may be in other respects quite healthy) will die shortly should there be no medical intervention. In this case the treatment can be considered to have a single objective (extension of life), and alternatives can be compared solely on that basis (e.g. Klarman *et al.*, 1968).

Perhaps more use could be made of these two simplifications, although both have associated problems. In the case of (a), are there many pairs of treatment alternatives where outcome in the two is roughly equivalent? In the varicose veins example it is now found that on the basis of six-year follow-up the more costly method is medically superior (Hobbs, 1974). In the case of (b), should one judge treatments merely on the basis of one aspect of their performance? In the chronic renal failure example one must ask whether one year of life gained by dialysis is equivalent to a year gained through transplantation. If one believes that they are not equivalent one may need a more detailed description of output in order to establish the appropriate trade-off between the outcomes produced by the two treatments. (In the study cited above, Klarman *et al.* (1968) assumed that one year of life gained by dialysis was equivalent to 0.75 years gained by transplantation.)

(iv) There are examples where, although a large NHS information system exists, the information collected is of little use in this type of evaluative work. The NHS hospital costing system is one such example. Partly because of the aggregate nature of the presentation of cost data, cost–benefit and cost effectiveness studies have run into practical difficulties in ascertaining the costs of particular health treatments. This is particularly true of those treatments carried out in hospitals. The movement away from the old 'subjective' cost headings and the presentation of hospital costs by specialty is likely to be of limited use since specialties themselves typically embrace a very heterogeneous set of treatments. There have been several attempts to obtain more detailed cost information (e.g. Babson, 1973; Russell, 1974). A comparison of these attempts suggests that the results obtained are highly dependent on the unavoidable (but nevertheless arbitrary) assumptions made (Mason *et al.*, 1973). Unfortunately, many cost–benefit analysts have treated these costing problems too lightly, and merely present cost data based on the average costs published in hospital cost returns.

(v) As far as one can tell, much (economic) evaluative work has been carried out by agencies or individuals *divorced* from the decision-making process. Exceptions to this would be those studies commissioned by the US Department of Health, Education and Welfare (e.g. Le Sourd *et al.*, 1968) and the Department of Health and Social Security (e.g. Gravelle, 1976; Adler *et al.*, 1974; Mills, 1976; Russell *et al.*, 1977). DHSS have also undertaken some studies of their own (e.g. Glass and Cove, 1976). Recently there appears to be some additional interest from clinicians who are concerned about the efficiency of their own treatments, but probably most studies have been undertaken by academic researchers who have no direct clinical or managerial responsibility for resource allocation decisions.

Perhaps the separation of evaluative work from the decision-making context may be one reason for there appearing to be little modification of existing practice as a result of the work undertaken so far. This phenomenon is not confined to economic evaluation. In a recent consultative document, DHSS feel it necessary to draw to one's attention forty 'Innovations in Clinical Practice', many of which date back to 1970 and before, that presumably have not yet gained wide practical application (DHSS, 1976a, pp. 34–7).

(vi) It must be remembered that evaluative studies themselves consume scarce resources. No actual estimates of this exist, although one expects the variance to be quite large, bearing in mind the differing degrees of sophistication of study-type.

5.4 'ALTERNATIVES' TO ECONOMIC EVALUATION

Sections 5.2 and 5.3 have argued the relevance of, and the state of the art in, economic evaluation in health care. It was seen that the cost–benefit approach (the approach used by economists to evaluate alternative health treatments) attempts to consider both the inputs (resources) used and the outputs produced by health treatments. Bearing in mind some of the technical problems outlined, potential alternatives deserve consideration. Here we discuss *input monitoring* and *medical evaluation*, since it is occasionally suggested that these give a guide to efficiency. However, it will be seen that they do not represent true alternatives to economic evaluation since neither considers both inputs and outputs.[6]

5.4.1 Input monitoring

(a) Quantity of inputs

The most common method of monitoring the quantity of inputs used in health treatments is through expenditure comparisons. For example, comparisons are often made of hospital cost per case or cost per inpatient week. Alternatively, comparisons may be made of the unit costs of (hospital) departmental service provision – cost per meal served, cost per 100 weighted pathology requests and so on.

The most obvious shortcoming of this approach to evaluation is that outputs are ignored. In evaluating the performance (say) of two hospitals, or in comparing two health treatments, one should require information not only of the resources consumed but also of the results produced.

(b) Quality of inputs

Monitoring the quality of inputs is really an indirect way of monitoring output. Examples of this approach are 'medical audit' or 'peer review', and hospital 'accreditation' schemes. One problem with such approaches is their supposition that 'good' inputs or 'good' processes generate 'good' outputs. Some evidence suggests that this is not necessarily the case (Brook and Appel, 1973). It may be that the notions of what is 'good' or 'adequate' (in the input sense) often derive from past habit or professional prejudice rather than from empirical estimation.[7] However, even if input quality were an adequate guide to output, it remains that output only is being considered.

5.4.2 Medical evaluation

It has already been noted (Section 5.2) that the estimation of the effectiveness of medical intervention is normally necessary to enable economic evaluation to be carried out. However, can the estimation of medical effectiveness alone provide one with a suitable framework for deciding upon what is the best use of resources? One could argue that the identification, and elimination, of ineffective treatments gives a guide to efficiency, since ineffective treatments will normally be inefficient too, as they consume scarce resources yet produce little of value to the community. Nevertheless, a major problem arises when, given the overall restriction on resources available for health care, it is necessary to choose between *effective* treatments. If the choice is (say) between two (mutually exclusive) alternative treatments for the same condition, is the more effective treatment to be chosen every time, regardless of relative cost? It may be that, when relative costs are taken into consideration, a decision taken in accordance with the efficiency criterion may result in the selection of the less effective (but less costly) treatment.[8] It should *not* be inferred from such a choice that to be more effective is not a 'good' thing. Merely it would imply that, given scarcity, the extra resources consumed by the more costly (but more effective) treatment could be used in other activities, generating a greater benefit to the community.

Therefore it is suggested that, unless one would be prepared to select the most effective treatment every time (regardless of relative effectiveness and relative cost), the assessment of medical effectiveness alone does not provide one with a sufficiently wide framework within which to decide upon the best use of resources.

5.5 ECONOMIC EVALUATION IN THE NHS – THE FUTURE

In this section the possibilities for economic evaluation within the NHS are set out. In suggesting how economic evaluation can be pursued, the existence of technical problems, particularly in the field of output measurement, is not denied. However, it has been indicated that some progress has been made in this area and that possibilities exist for circumventing some of the output measurement problems, provided that it is possible to restrict the scope of the analysis (i.e. to choices between alternative methods of fulfilling a particular, predetermined, objective). Also, the decisions to which these technical problems relate are at present being taken on the basis of less accurate or less comprehensive information than would be provided by the evaluative procedures proposed.

An important aspect of the suggestions made below is that they offer opportunities for the closer integration of economic evaluation and health service decision-making. In so far as the criterion of economic efficiency is important in deciding upon the best use of resources, it is preferable that those evaluations carried out are relevant to the health service resource allocation decisions being made.

Two possible opportunities for the development of economic evaluation have been identified:

(i) *In the clinical assessment of new medical treatments.* Most new treatments are likely to be medically evaluated. Bearing in mind the dependence of economic evaluation on parameters estimated through medical evaluation, the performance of medical evaluation presents a good opportunity for further development as economic evaluation.[9] The use of economic evaluation would ensure that new treatments were being assessed not only in terms of their medical effect but also in terms of their cost relative to treatments in current use. This is important since recent trends in medicine have not been towards less sophisticated and less expensive procedures. There would be a particularly strong case for economic appraisal where the adoption of the new treatment is likely to bring about large changes in resource-utilisation.

One must recognise the lead taken by the DHSS in the undertaking and commissioning of economic evaluations of new treatments and procedures. These were noted in Section 5.3.2. The DHSS initiatives have the advantage that, where a new treatment is likely to be adopted all over the country, a single evaluation may suffice, and the scarce resources required for such evaluative procedures can be used economically. However, such centralised initiatives do have the problem that local circumstances differ within the NHS and what is efficient in one location may not be so in another.[10] Also there is the more general problem of inducing local agencies to act on the basis of centrally commissioned research. The central agency must decide whether local agencies are merely to be informed of the results of the research, whether financial inducements in the form (say) of special grants are to be offered, or whether a directive is to be issued. Therefore, although the DHSS initiatives are to be welcomed, the possibilities for economic evaluation at other levels in the system should be explored.

(ii) *In the NHS planning system.* The planning system would appear to be the most appropriate home for on-going economic evaluation at all levels in the NHS.

The underlying purpose of all planning in the NHS is to seek to achieve the most efficient and cost-effective use of all available resources for the benefit of those who use the service. [DHSS, 1976b, para. 3.6]

Also, evaluation in the context of the planning system would not be restricted merely to new treatments but would also apply to existing treatments and procedures.[11]

The DHSS clearly recognise this possibility:

In planning for the most effective and efficient use of resources, it is essential that there should be a willingness to subject traditional methods of delivering services to critical reappraisal. [DHSS, 1976b, para. 2.9]

However, despite the acknowledged need for economic evaluation within the planning system, one does not (as yet) detect any extensive employment of the methods of economic appraisal outlined in Section 5.3. There are a number of possible explanations for this.

(a) *Lack of economic expertise.* One would expect there to be few staff within the NHS with the expertise necessary to carry out such evaluative work. Therefore, if economic evaluation were to be encouraged there would be a need for more personnel to be trained in the relevant techniques.

(b) *Lack of evaluative information.* It has already been indicated that, where information systems do exist, the information collected may be of little evaluative use (e.g. the cost data collected routinely through the NHS hospital costing system). Furthermore, some information relevant to evaluative studies is not normally collected at all, e.g. those data relating to the use of patients' resources in health treatments and those relating to the output of health treatments. Also, other relevant data, such as those relating to resource use in health treatments by other public bodies, may be collected but will not often be available to the health service decision-maker.

(c) *Lack of incentives.* It may be that local agencies are uncertain of the likely pay-off from employing evaluative procedures, particularly as the procedures themselves consume scarce resources. Also, within the present budgeting arrangements, there is little direct incentive for NHS agencies to behave efficiently. For instance, in attempting to maximise the quantity of care provided, or even the resultant output from that care, the health services manager will be concerned mainly with such a maximisation as constrained by the resources (i.e. budget) placed at his disposal. He is less likely to be concerned with the effects of his actions on the budgets of other public organisations or private households, since such consideration is unlikely to be 'rewarded' within a budgetary system that is concerned with controlling expenditure within the various agencies providing health care, rather than with minimising the cost of a given health care programme to the community as a whole. Therefore, he may have little incentive to use a decision-making tool such as cost–benefit analysis which attempts to appraise alternative courses of action through a consideration of costs and benefits falling on, or accruing to, *all* members of the community.

(d) *Other difficulties in integrating economic evaluation into health service decision-making.* These may include difficulties in undertaking economic appraisals with sufficient speed to enable planning deadlines to be met. It may be that, for shorter planning horizons only, studies of lower levels of sophistication can be undertaken. Of course, one reason for the lack of quick answers is that much of the relevant information will have to be collected by the analyst, since it is not available routinely.

It is likely that a combination of most of these factors is in evidence. Therefore it is suggested that there is a need to examine in more detail the scope for, and the operation of, economic evaluation at various levels within the NHS. In particular, answers to the following questions will be required.

(i) What would economic evaluation contribute to decision-making at each level in view of the constraints (e.g. the 'deadlines' imposed by the planning process, and the scarce resources required for the undertaking of evaluation)?

(ii) What are the information needs for such evaluative procedures?

(iii) Do evaluative data need to be collected on a routine basis?

(iv) Are we likely to require more data in total, or can these data be viewed as a substitute for some of the data collected at present?

(v) What incentives are required to induce local agencies to behave efficiently?

(vi) Can these incentives be incorporated within the existing budgetary system?

(vii) If economic evaluation were to be undertaken at the local level, how could the relevant skills best be obtained?

It is obvious that the expansion of economic evaluation within the NHS, particularly through the planning system, would require careful thought. However, it is argued that, if the criterion of economic efficiency *is* considered to be important in deciding upon the best use of resources, then a closer integration between economic evaluation and decision-making (difficult though that may be) is to be encouraged. The alternative would be a continuation of the present arrangements which represent the worst of both worlds. On the one hand scarce resources are being consumed in undertaking evaluative work that, with the exception of some of those studies commissioned by DHSS, is likely to bring about little change in NHS operation; on the other hand the vast majority of resource allocation decisions within the NHS are being undertaken without thorough and explicit consideration of the criterion of economic efficiency.

5.6   CONCLUDING REMARKS

(i) It has been argued that the criterion of economic efficiency (which implies the use of available resources so as to generate the largest possible social benefit) is essential in the consideration of the best use of resources. Also, it has been argued that economic evaluation provides a better framework for choice between health service alternatives than many other procedures (such as input monitoring and medical evaluation).

(ii) Economic evaluation is generally reliant upon the assessment of the medical effectiveness of treatments, and therefore advocacy of economic evaluation further implies advocacy of medical evaluation.

(iii) A review of economic evaluative work in the health field shows that progress has been made but that some technical problems still exist, particularly in the difficult areas of output measurement and valuation. Some of these problems can be avoided provided that one is prepared to restrict the analysis merely to choices between alternative ways of meeting the same treatment objective, rather than to the wider question of choice between objectives themselves. In any case, the decisions to which the technical problems relate are at the moment being undertaken on the basis of less accurate or less comprehensive information than evaluative studies would provide.

(iv) Much evaluative work to date has been carried out by those not directly concerned with health service decision-making. It is argued that if economic efficiency is a relevant criterion then more integration between analysis and decision-making would be desirable.

(v) Two possible opportunities for such an integration have been discussed: (a) in the evaluation of new medical treatments, and (b) within the NHS planning system.

NOTES

1. The author is grateful to J. Wiseman and R. Sugden, in addition to the other contributors to this volume, for comments on earlier drafts. Acknowledgement is made to SSRC, who have provided financial support for a study of the cost effectiveness of health treatments.

2. 'Scarcity' in this context relates not to the existence of a governmental budget constraint on the resources devoted to health care, but rather to the more fundamental notion that there will never be enough resources to satisfy human wants completely. We can view the former as a practical reminder of the latter. The use of scarce resources in one activity means that the opportunity to use them in another is forgone.

3. Where the value of resources (or cost) reflects their value to the community in their best alternative use.

4. In practice, this theoretical position may not always be upheld. Some economists feel that other values may be used when (for instance) there is considerable consumer ignorance about the product. (Some argue this in the case of health care.) However, values from other sources (such as policy-makers) are often used merely because they are more easily obtainable.

5. In the example above it would be possible to give the families of clients a grant (or tax relief) for caring for the elderly at home.

6. The necessity to consider both inputs and outputs is perhaps more apparent when we remember that the resources consumed by a particular health treatment (given scarcity) represent outputs forgone elsewhere.

7. There may be other reasons for encouraging schemes such as 'peer review'. For instance, it is possible that such schemes can encourage a useful dialogue between clinicians in aspects of their clinical work. However, they should not be viewed as a substitute for full medical or economic evaluation.

8. If the two treatments were equally effective, then presumably all would agree that the less costly (most cost-effective) treatment be chosen.

9. The integration of economic and medical evaluation is most relevant when the medical evaluation being performed is of the 'pragmatic' type (Schwartz and Lellouch, 1967). 'Pragmatic' medical evaluation aims at making a decision between therapies, whereas 'explanatory' medical evaluation aims merely at acquiring information on the effects of the treatments.

10. Nevertheless, by careful reading of a good evaluative study, representatives of local agencies should be able to tell whether or not local circumstances are likely to alter the study's general conclusions with regard to efficiency.

11. It is worth noting that some believe that many existing treatments have not been *medically* evaluated, let alone *economically* evaluated (Cochrane, 1972).

REFERENCES

Acton, J. P. (1973) *Evaluating Public Programs to Save Lives: The Case of Heart Attacks* Santa Monica, California, Rand Corporation, R-950-RC.

Acton, J. P. (1975) *Measuring the Social Impact of Heart and Circulatory Disease Programs: Preliminary Framework and Estimates* Santa Monica, California, Rand Corporation, R-1697-NHLI.

Adler, M. W. *et al.* (1974) 'A Randomised Controlled Trial of Early Discharge for Inguinal Hernia and Varicose Veins – Some Problems of Methodology' *Medical Care* vol. 12, no. 6, pp. 541–7.

Babson, J. (1973) *Disease Costing*, Manchester University Press.

Brook, R. H. and Appel, F. A. (1973) 'Quality of Care Assessment: Choosing a Method of Peer Review' *New England Journal of Medicine* June, pp. 1323–9.

Bush, J. W., Chen, M. M. and Patrick, D. L. (1973) 'Health Status Index in Cost Effectiveness: Analysis of a PKU Program' in Berg (ed.), *Health Status Indexes* Chicago, Hospital Research and Educational Trust.

Cochrane. A. L. (1972) *Effectiveness and Efficiency: Random Reflections on Health Services* London, Nuffield Provincial Hospitals Trust.

DHSS (1976a) *Priorities for Health and Personal Social Services in England: A Consultative Document* London, HMSO.

DHSS (1976b) *The NHS Planning System* June, London, HMSO.

Drummond, M. F. (1976) 'The Costs and Benefits of Alternative Health Treatments' paper delivered to the Health Economists' Study Group, York, July 1976.

Glass, N. J. and Cove, A. R. (1976) 'Economic Consequences for the Public Sector of a Spina Bifida Screening Programme' mimeo, London, DHSS.

Gravelle, H. S. E. (1976) 'The Economic Evaluation of Screening for Breast Cancer: a Tentative Methodology' paper delivered to Health Economists' Study Group, York, July 1976.

Hobbs, J. T. (1974) 'Surgery and Sclerotherapy in the Treatment of Varicose Veins: a Random Trial,' *Archs. Surg.* vol. 109, pp. 793–6.

Jones-Lee, M. W. (1976) *The Value of Life: An Economic Analysis* London, Martin Robertson.

Klarman, H. E., Francis, J. O'S and Rosenthal, G. D. (1968) 'Cost-Effectiveness Analysis Applied to the Treatment of Chronic Renal Failure', *Medical Care* vol. 6, pp. 48–54.

Le Sourd, D. A. *et al.* (1968) *Benefit–Cost analysis of Kidney Disease Programs* Public Health Service Publication No. 1941, Washington, DC, Department of Health, Education and Welfare.

Mason, A. M. S., Perry, J. A. and Skegg, J. L. (1973) 'Disease Costing in Hospitals: A Review of Completed Work' Introductory paper for a one-day symposium to be held at Northwick Park Hospital (mimeo).

Mills, M. (1976) *The Application of Cost–Benefit Analysis to Health Services – Some Problems Raised by an Evaluation of Flexible Fibreoptic Endoscopes* Research Paper Series, Public Sector Economics Research Centre, University of Leicester.

Piachaud, D. and Weddell, J. M. (1972) 'The Economics of Treating Varicose Veins' *Int. J. Epidemiology* vol. 1, no. 3, pp. 287–94.

Pole, J. D. (1971) 'Mass Radiography: a Cost–Benefit Approach' in G. McLachlan (ed.) *Problems and Progress in Medical Care – 5th Series* London, Nuffield Provincial Hospitals Trust.

Rosser, R. M. and Watts, V. C. (1972) 'The Measurement of Hospital Output' *Int. J. Epidemiology* vol. 1, no. 4, pp. 361–8.

Rosser, R. M. and Watts, V. C. (1974) 'The Development of a Classification of Symptoms of Sickness and its Use to Measure the Output of a Hospital' in D. Lees and S. Shaw (eds), *Impairment, Disability and Handicap* London, Heinemann for SSRC.

Royal Commission on the National Health Service (1976) *The Task of the Commission* London, HMSO.

Russell, E. M. (1974) *Patient Costing Study* Scottish Health Services Studies No. 31 Edinburgh, Scottish Home and Health Department.

Russell, I. T. *et al.* (1977) 'Day Case Surgery for Hernias and Haemorrhoids: a Clinical, Social and Economic Evaluation' *The Lancet* pp. 844–7.

Schwartz, D. and Lellouch, J. (1967) 'Explanatory and Pragmatic Attitudes in Therapeutic Trials' *J. Chron. Dis.* vol. 20, pp. 637–48.

Torrance, G. W., Sackett, D. L. and Thomas, W. H. (1973) 'Utility Maximisation Model for Program Evaluation: a Demonstration Application' in R. L. Berg (ed), *Health Status Indexes* Chicago, Hospital Research and Educational Trust.

Wager, R. (1972) *Care of the Elderly – an Exercise in Cost–Benefit Analysis Commissioned by Essex County Council* London, IMTA.

Williams, A. H. (1974) 'The Cost–Benefit Approach' *British Medical Bulletin* vol. 30, no. 3 (September), pp. 252–6.

6. The Budget as a (Mis-)Information System

Alan Williams[1]

Budgets serve many purposes. The most widely known is that of cash control (who is spending how much on what, and with whose authority?). The information deriving from that process is commonly used to forecast cash requirements; to set financial targets ('we really must try to do better than just break even next year'); and, in a limited sense, to monitor the performance of those with budget responsibilities.

With increased emphasis on planning, there is immediately brought to light a serious deficiency in the existing data base (and in the information system that generates it). When it comes to telling us about the efficiency with which existing resources are deployed, and on potentially better ways of deploying them, it is tempting to try to make good this deficiency by turning to the budgeting system for the missing information. It is on the dangers of uncritical use of this information that I shall concentrate in this paper.

In a recent paper on the problems of monitoring performance in the health service, Sir Richard Doll has expressed scepticism about the extent to which it is possible to be vigorous and systematic in this difficult field (yet making it clear that he was sympathetic to such endeavours). He epitomised his position as being one in which he believed that this was a field in which 'gardening is real, but botany is bogus'.[2] It is on that telling analogy that I have structured this essay, in the hope that by so doing I can demonstrate that, if we are ever to break out of the limitations of gardener's folklore, we do need a strong dose of botanical knowledge.

6.1 CLEARING THE GROUND

Any rational planning process must provide for the following five elements:

(i) the *recording* of the decisions that have been made (so that those who made the decisions shall be clear about what they decided, and why, and what they expect to happen as a result);

(ii) the *transmission* of key information about these decisions to those who have to carry them out (since it is rarely the case that implementation requires actions only on the part of those who are parties to the decisions in the first place);

(iii) the *monitoring* of performance (which means organising the collection and feedback of selected information about what actually happened in terms that relate to the intentions of decision-makers);

(iv) the *evaluation* of outcomes (i.e. the judgement as to whether what happened is better or worse than what was intended, and, if different, why, and what, if anything, should be done differently next time);

(v) a fresh round of *decision* (which may simply be to repeat the decision made last time; but may, at the other extreme, involve a radical re-thinking of objectives and policies in a particular area, entailing cessation of activity).

At this point the cycle would be repeated, and in some complex situations (iii) and (iv) might be going on continuously alongside (i) and (ii), with (v) feeding in only sporadically. In some routine-hidden situations, (v) does not really exist because the system has so much momentum it can tick over anyway so long as the external environment remains stable and accommodating, hence no need is seen for (iii) and (iv); 'planning', in my understanding of the term, is absent (and, some would argue, unnecessary).

Before entering the main arena of discussion, there are two other basic notions that need to be introduced. The first is the distinction between an organisation and an activity, and the second is the difference between input, throughput and output.

An 'organisation' is here taken to mean any legal–administrative entity that has a recognisable corporate identity (e.g. a hospital, or a GP's practice, or the X-ray department of a hospital, or the DHSS). An activity, on the other hand, is some task-orientated grouping of resources, defined by what they are doing rather than what they are or to whom they belong (e.g. diagnosing illness, or alleviating poverty or providing meals for the elderly). Sometimes one particular organisation will carry out many (narrowly defined) activities; sometimes one particular (broadly defined) activity will require the collaboration of many organisations; and sometimes (but all too rarely) an organisation and an activity will exactly coincide. The general non-coincidence of organisations and activities will prove to be a major source of difficulty for us, because it is broadly the case that budgets relate to organisations, but plans relate to activities.

By 'input' is meant the resources used in an activity or organisation. By 'output' is meant what has been achieved, in terms related to the objectives of the activity or organisation, be those objectives (or outputs) tangible or intangible. For instance, the 'input' of teachers disseminating information about personal hygiene into the activity of teaching children in school might yield an 'output' of reduced gastro-intestinal infection. Output, like objectives, can be articulated at different levels of generality. To take the latter example a bit further, it might be said that 'reduced gastro-intestinal infection' is only an 'intermediate' output, the 'final' output being an increase in life expectation free of pain and disability. Going back in the other direction, the extent of teachers' knowledge about personal hygiene will itself be an 'output' from some training programme, etc. The general point is that, whether a particular element is input or output is relative to a specified focus of interest. Once that is defined, matters should fall into place. This still leaves us with one other definitional matter, the measure of work done (e.g. numbers of children taught), which is neither input nor output; and it is that which I shall call 'throughput'.

6.2   RECOGNISING WEEDS

Some recent correspondence in *The Times* on the alleged efficacy of talking lovingly to plants as a means of stimulating healthy growth led one disgruntled contributor to express disbelief in the whole notion on the grounds that his intemperate abuse of weeds over many years did not seem to have stunted their growth in the slightest! A later correspondent was then moved to suggest that perhaps a weed was, in essence, a plant impervious to insults. So, it seems, is the case with traditional budgets, which I shall now caricature in a slightly unfair but, I am sure, readily recognisable manner.

The traditional budget has three typical characteristics: it is annual; it is concerned solely with inputs; and it relates essentially to those inputs for which cash is required. Its 'annualness' is probably a cultural hangover from the time when we were primarily an agrarian society, and when the annual cycle of seasons was the dominant feature of all activities (this fits well, of course, with gardeners' folklore). Its survival has been reinforced by legal and administrative routines in parliamentary and statutory provisions, but is of dubious relevance in a planning context. I shall not consider it in depth here, because it is peripheral to my main theme, but it does introduce some distortions in information flow which we cannot ignore.

The input orientation, and especially its cash connotations, can best be epitomised by rehearsing the processes that this kind of budgeting generates when we go through the five elements set out above. The *recording* of decisions tends to be a list of sums of money allocated to particular agencies (organisations) to be spent on particular inputs (e.g. so much for wages and salaries, so much for supplies, so much for fuel, etc.). The information *transmitted* tends to be a schedule of spending authorisations, in which a person is told what he has to spend on what items over what space of time (and this is frequently all he is told – he may not know what others have to spend, or what he is supposed to be achieving with his spendings). *Monitoring* consists of keeping a running tally of how much has been spent under each head (plus, in the more sophisticated systems, how much has been committed, and how this compares with previous years' patterns and with the current allocations), and this may or may not be fed back to the budget-holder on a continuous basis with appropriate words of encouragement or admonition. *Evaluation* essentially comprises the comparison of estimates with 'outturn', and if the latter exceeds the former by a sizable margin all sorts of 'tut-tutting' will occur, accompanied by varying degrees of inquisitorial beastliness. If the figures are exactly equal, the books obviously need auditing to see where the spare cash is being stashed away or where the overspendings have been concealed. If the outturn falls far short of the estimate, you suspect that you were taken for a ride at estimate time and sack the budget-holder for unprofessional practice! *Decision* then consists of trimming the margins here and there, but allowing a general overall drift in line with the change in total available. Perhaps this is why it has recently become the vogue to refer to 'forward' planning, to distinguish it presumably from old-fashioned 'backward' planning, the basic ethic of which was 'to he that hath much, shall more be given: but from him that hath something left over, shall be taken away even that which he hath!' Hence the proud claim of the astute financial gamesman, 'Never knowingly underspent'.

My prime purpose is not, however, to poke gentle fun at (or, as some might see it, to make cheap gibes at the expense of) traditional financial control systems. My more serious purpose is to test it out as an information source for planning purposes. It seems reasonable, for instance, to expect it to answer the question, 'What does X cost?', where X is a unit of activity, measured preferably in output terms but, failing that, at least in throughput terms. For instance, we might reasonably ask how much it costs to get a man with a hernia working normally again, or what it costs to check whether a pale listless patient has anaemia. In fact, it is currently impossible to answer those questions, except by painstaking research, and the reasons for this are well worth exploring.

In the first place, no one has had any great incentive to find out, since the organisations responsible for (different parts of) the activities mentioned do not think like that, do not plan like that, are not controlled like that and do not run like that. So 'managers' have had no reason to devote scarce resources to collecting that kind of information. Secondly, even if we asked them more limited questions, about what it costs to carry out their bit of the overall activity (say the inpatient treatment of the man with a hernia), they will have a job disentangling the hernia cases from the others, they will only know about the costs that show up in their budgets, and even then they will probably only be able to tell you what the average costs are over all cases treated, and not the incremental costs of a typical additional case. These are serious shortcomings from a planning viewpoint, because we shall usually not be considering an increase in all types of case equally, and it will rarely be true that all relevant resources will show up in the 'manager's' budget (e.g. the use of space, or of patients' time, or of various associated services provided 'free' by other organisations), or that there are no fixed costs (or economies of scale) so that the distinction between 'average' and 'incremental' costs would cease to be important.

A classic case of this sort has arisen over the pressure to reduce length of stay in hospitals. Some estimates of cost savings have concentrated on the average cost per occupied bed-day (i.e. total hospital costs divided by total number of occupied bed-days). On this basis, reducing length of stay by 10 per cent reduces costs by 10 per cent. But since the costliest parts of treatment are typically concentrated in the earlier parts of an episode of impatient treatment, the days 'saved' are much 'cheaper' than the 'average' day, hence average costs represent gross over-estimates of potential savings. Moreover, if bed occupancy rates are kept up by admitting more patients (i.e. increasing 'throughput'), although cost per 'case' will fall, cost per occupied bed-day will rise, since a larger proportion of the 'days' are 'expensive' days). More serious still, however, is the way 'cost per case' has slipped into the act, for it should really be 'hospital cost per episode of inpatient treatment', since there is no guarantee that it is not the same 'case' coming in and out several times, and in any case 'inpatient' episodes are usually linked with outpatient consultations before and/or after the inpatient episode itself, and the costs of these are not included. Moreover, the patients' costs are being ignored in all this, as are the costs falling on non-hospital health services, local authority social services, voluntary bodies, and friends and relatives who provide support. Thus, if we rely on our cash-orientated input budget for hospitals as the major source of information on costs for planning purposes (even with respect to hospitals), we are likely to be grossly misled by the information it generates, unless we are aware of its inherent defects and take pains to make them good.

Thus my summary judgement on traditional budgeting is that its prime defect is its *input* orientation, and its secondary defect that it does not even count *all* the inputs. But is it possible to conceive anything better?

6.3 SOWING SEEDS

If we are to break out of this situation we need to have budgets related to objectives (output budgeting) or, as a step in that direction, to activities that have clear objectives (programme budgeting). Thus 'organisations' are not given pride of place, but are left to establish their role (if any!) in relation to the objectives/activities that are being promoted by the budget-holders. This apparently simple conceptual change has far-reaching implications.

In the first place, it forces people to think about objectives, and where they fit into the order of things (a botanical rather than a gardening question). It also enables those controlling the system to ask whether there ought not to be brought into existence some organisations or activities that do not currently exist; and although one *could* rely on random mutation and natural selection to generate the required evolutionary adaptation to changing circumstances, a little botanical knowledge about hybridisation possibilities and a policy of deliberate interbreeding might speed the process up a bit.

The practical manifestations of this change in budgeting philosophy would be that we would have, as primary budget-holders, directors of agencies concerned, say, with the welfare of the elderly, or of children, or of some similar 'client group', who would then 'buy in' services from 'activity' agencies (e.g. those providing home helps, domiciliary nursing, residential care, medical attention of various kinds, etc.). These 'activity' agencies will normally be providing services for more than one 'client group' agency (e.g. home helps will be provided for maternity or acute and chronic medical cases for groups other than the elderly), so problems of cost apportionment and appropriate reimbursement mechanisms will immediately arise. These difficult problems are held out as reasons for sticking with a system that does not 'generate' such problems. Yet it is precisely the failure of the existing system to grapple effectively with these problems that underlies its weaknesses as an information system for planning purposes. It is not that the problems are not there; it is rather that they are not confronted.

That the gardener's life would be more uncomfortable under the watchful eye of the critical botanist cannot be denied, but he should perhaps be made to pay that price if sufficient good comes out of it. Returning to the planning process set out above, let us see how it would now look. The *recording* of the decision would be more like a 'contract' between the buying agency and the selling agency, whereby the latter is not just told how much it will be 'paid', but also what services it is to deliver in return. The *transmission* of this information will similarly need to include both expected 'output' or 'activity' levels as well as expected remuneration for inputs used. *Monitoring* will, similarly, range over both output and input, so that *evaluation* can take the form of cost effectiveness studies, and not just cost comparisons. In this way the higher-level agency would have a sensible basis for reviewing its decisions on the next round, by shifting resources towards those agencies that are proving relatively more cost-effective *in terms of the high level agency's objectives*.

There is still one weakness in this alternative view of the world that needs to be put right, namely the failure of agencies to report costs that do not fall on their budgets. This is a very serious and pervasive problem throughout the economic system, and the solution obviously lies in finding some way of incorporating these notional (or 'shadow') costs into budgeting processes. One simple radical way of doing this is to make the agency actually pay for the resource in question (e.g., patients are paid for the time they have to wait after the appointed time for a consultation). If that is considered too strong a dose of weedkiller for initial applications, then as a more moderate (and probably less effective) start we could use sample 'audits' of such waiting times to estimate 'hidden' costs of various agencies, and simply use these when it comes to the monitoring and evaluation phase of the planning process. Again, I do not under-estimate the conceptual and practical difficulties of establishing such 'shadow' costs; but it is no excuse for not grappling with them to say that the current budgeting system has the advantage that you don't have to bother with such niceties. . . . I would rather say that the current budgeting system has the 'advantage' that it has systematically obscured such gross inefficiencies!

6.4 STIMULATING HEALTHY GROWTH

Defenders of the present system will doubtless feel that it has been pilloried unjustly, and that I am giving insufficient credit to the recent developments in hospital costing that have manifested a steady movement away from a sporadic, local, unco-ordinated assembly of financial data based solely on broad input categories. By linking such data to hospital activity analysis, it becomes possible to cost out particular services over departments, and hence move the system in the direction of 'activity' budgets.

The difficulty here is the difference in focus between short-term 'managerial' considerations and long-term 'planning' considerations. For the former, it is confusing and irritating to the head of a department to have 'loaded' on to his budget items over which he feels he has no control (like a fixed percentage of the institution's total heating bill, or an imputed rental for the space he uses, or a share of central administrative overheads). What he wants is information only about the items that are susceptible to day-to-day or week-to-week 'management', and that is all that those monitoring his performance in context need to concentrate on.

When it comes to reviewing the overall scale of the activity in a planning context, however, we are going to need data on those variables that lie outside short-term managerial discretion, but that could become possible objects for adjustment. Since hospital costing activity has (perhaps properly) been focused primarily on the former set of problems and not on the latter, it cannot be held up as an answer to my strictures, though it could be cited as evidence that the system is capable of healthy growth.

One fundamental limitation on such growth remains, however, and that is the notion that budgeting is 'treasurer's business'. In the old-fashioned sense, it was. In this broader sense it is not, because once budgeting is openly and inextricably intertwined with objective setting, priorities, performance targets set in non-financial terms and monitoring and evaluation in the broadest sense, it is essentially a multi-disciplinary process. Apart from economists and administrators, too little serious study and *informed* criticism of budgeting processes has been forthcoming from the other professional groups in the health service, which may partly explain their current frustrations. While the mystique of medicine has come under severe attack, the mystique of accountancy has hardly been touched. If this reappraisal is to be conducted in a constructive way, then it needs to be made clear what each contributes to the process, and in a system of output or programme budgeting there is a very clear and central role for the non-financial information, whereas the traditional budget is simply finance, finance and still more finance. So in broadening our conceptual thinking, we also increase our capability to take on board new knowledge.

Here I return to the main theme. For me, evolution connotes accidental adaptation through unco-ordinated innovations. It has got us broadly where we are today (like it or not). With luck it will see us through tomorrow. Planning connotes deliberate adaptation through co-ordinated innovation. It has had some spectacular results (like them or not) in the last few centuries. With good judgement (and a little luck) it will ensure that tomorrow's world is a better place. Put starkly, then, the choice seems to be between gardening as best we can with what nature provides, or setting up a laboratory blueprint based on the best that the botanical sciences can offer. But even within this (by now rather strained) analogy, there is a middle way, viz., to adopt as our model the botanical garden. The objective then becomes to improve on nature in a scientific but realistically sustainable way (the plants will grow and survive, often outside their natural habitats).

Thus, what we seem to need in our approach to budgets is a planning tool in the health service. Let us try transplanting some promising 'stock' which has all the theoretical (i.e. genetic) properties we need, so as to convert our present rather weedy growth into something we could be proud of. Why be content with a scruffy suburban allotment when you could make a play for Kew Gardens?

NOTES

1. This paper is a revised version of a talk originally delivered to the Association of Health Service Treasurers on 14 February 1974.
2. Doll, Richard (1973) 'Monitoring the National Health Service' (*Proceedings of the Royal Society of Medicine*, vol. 66, pp. 729–40.

PART III

Finance

7.   Prices and the Demand for Care

J. A. Cairns and M. C. Snell[1]

7.1   INTRODUCTION

Pricing in the health services is an emotive issue, and one where it is often difficult to distinguish the arguments and basic value judgements involved. One common starting point for examining the issues in pricing for health care is that resources should be allocated to those people and in those fields where society most wishes them to be used, and it is with this viewpoint in mind that we examine in Section 7.2 arguments for and against the imposition of charges for health care. In particular, we look at possible aims of a health service, and examine whether zero-prices, as those most frequently used for NHS services, are logically consistent with these aims, as well as assessing whether other prices might fulfil these aims more easily. In Section 7.3 we consider how the demand for various health services is affected by changes in price. We also examine the effects on consumers' demand for health care of introducing a price system, and the differential impact of pricing between income groups.

7.2   ISSUES

Proponents of pricing argue for the use of a price system on the grounds that it allocates resources to those uses that individuals value most highly. Under a pricing system, an individual would not seek treatment unless its value to him was at least as high as the price he had to pay for it. If the price charged for any treatment were to be equal to the cost of treating an additional patient, no individual would receive care unless his valuation of that care were greater than the cost of providing it. The existence of any excess demand in such circumstances would suggest that some individuals currently not obtaining treatment would be willing to pay the cost of supplying additional treatments. Such an excess demand might be eliminated either by raising the price or by increasing supply. Thus, when a price for

95

a particular treatment is set at a level that equals the cost of treatment and also generates no excess demand, even the consumer who values it the least places a value on the treatment that is not less than its cost (or the value other individuals put upon the resources used). Given the limited resources in the economy, careful use of pricing can therefore allocate resources to those uses that individuals value most highly.

The pricing mechanism outlined above works on the basis that an individual compares his own valuation of receiving a particular treatment with the cost (to him) of that treatment. If his valuation is less than the cost he will not seek the treatment. However, if other members of society are affected by the health status of the individual and hence also value his receipt of that treatment, then it can be argued, even if he had decided not to seek the treatment himself, that if the total valuation (his plus everyone else's) of his receiving the treatment is greater than its cost (to society), he ought to receive treatment. We might say that society believes the individual 'needs' treatment. In this paper, a need for health care is said to exist when the sum of each individual's valuation of the delivery of that care exceeds the cost to society of delivering it.[2]

If other individuals are prepared to give up some part of their own income in order that another individual might consume more health care, it seems clear that society would benefit if such a transfer took place. We must ask firstly how such a transfer would best be organised and secondly whether it should be in cash or kind. One possible solution to the organisational problem is the formation of charities, and the widespread prewar existence of charities in the health field can undoubtedly be attributed to this collective feeling. However, a strong case can be made for the government itself acting as an agent for the whole population in its concerns of this kind, essentially superseding private action as a kind of national 'super-charity'. One benefit of government organisation derives from the conditional nature of much private giving (i.e. the amount one is willing to contribute for any particular purpose may depend on how much others are willing to give). Compulsory taxation may be an imperfect, but none the less a more efficient, response than voluntary financing.

If governmental action is deemed the appropriate method for redistribution, it must be decided whether the government should make transfer payments to low-income groups, thus enabling them to afford the health care society has decided they need, or make health care available free of charge (or at some price less than cost) to such groups. One's answer depends on a number of factors, not the least of which is one's value judgements. One may argue in favour of the income transfer, on the grounds that it would permit maximum freedom of choice. Alternatively, one may be less willing to give responsibility for choice to the recipients, believing that some other group of individuals has better knowledge of the level of health care that individuals ought to consume.

If the transfer takes the form of income, any part (including none) can be expended on health care, and therefore the benefit of the transfer to the donor could be relatively low per pound transferred. (While it is true that the benefit as perceived by the recipient will be higher, the donor's willingness-to-transfer may be lower.) If the decision to redistribute is a result of concern for individuals' health states and their consumption of health care, then redistribution in kind might be preferable. On the other hand, if the decision to redistribute results from concern about the income level of certain individuals rather than their health state, the income transfer would appear appropriate.

What we have termed 'redistribution in kind' can take a number of forms, such as the subsidisation of insurance premiums or of the price at point of contact, or the use of health vouchers that could be exchanged only for health care. Their identifying characteristic is that the redistribution does not simply give the individual increased command over all goods and services, but (to a greater or lesser extent) embodies restrictions on how he can 'spend' the transfer.

In the NHS, with few exceptions, health care is zero-priced. It has been suggested (Culyer, 1976) that the rationale for such a policy derives from the kind of argument we have outlined above. It is pertinent to ask why zero-pricing is used rather than other policy options, such as subsidised premiums. In general, in the NHS we have zero-prices not for certain user-groups but for all. Such universal zero pricing denies pricing any role in the allocation of health care among consumers. At least two general arguments can be identified in support of such a position, the first of which does not accept the benefits of pricing, and the second of which suggests why zero-pricing may be preferable to the other policy options.

Firstly, the valuations used to allocate health care under a price system are based on individuals' willingness-to-pay. Because the amount an individual is *willing* to pay will depend to some extent on the amount an individual is *able* to pay, greater weight will be put on the views of those with more wealth; also, different distributions of income may generate different valuations by the community of different forms of care. If the existing distribution of income is not the 'preferred' one, then the particular valuations it 'reveals' may be of little interest.

The other major argument for the universal zero-pricing of health care is based on the benefits of zero-pricing and the costs of selective pricing. It is argued that positive prices will deter some individuals from demanding care, the receipt of which would have a value to society in excess of its cost. The lower the price, the smaller will be the number of people deterred from seeking needed treatment. If we knew the price at which each individual would demand each treatment, it might be possible to ensure that each individual sought needed treatment by charging every individual a different price for each treatment so that use of a price mechanism might still appear attractive. However, we do not have the relevant information and the costs of obtaining it and of administering such a system would appear to be very high. If we believed that the deterrent effect of pricing was inversely related to the income of the individual, then we might approximate the desired outcome by charging different income *groups* different prices. A crude version of such a pricing system exists in the field of dental care in the United Kingdom. The choice of a universal zero-price may therefore be justified on the grounds that it may be the most cost-effective policy.

It is important to realise, that a zero price does not imply that everyone whom society feels ought to demand care will actually demand care. The most important reasons for this are that the individual faces costs of obtaining care, even in the absence of charges, and the fact that individuals differ as regards their preferences and knowledge. When seeking and undergoing treatment, the individual will forgo opportunities to engage in other activities such as work (paid or unpaid) or some form of leisure. Individuals will differ over the extent of their medical knowledge, such as the possible implications of certain symptoms, and as a result individuals with similar symptoms may make different decisions on seeking care. Some individuals may prefer to put up with a certain complaint rather than to undergo treatment, or they may simply choose to be less healthy than others. For all these reasons it is the case that some individuals may seek care only if faced by a negative price, that is, if paid to visit a doctor.

When money prices are zero there is likely to be an excess demand for health care, as evidenced in the NHS by the length of time one may wait for a consultation with a GP or for admission to a hospital. Some form of rationing must exist to decide who gets priority. At present, rationing is carried out largely by doctors, each with reference to his own particular concept of medical need. Thus, if we are to argue that zero-pricing enables treatment to be given to those whom society decides need it, then doctors should interpret and act on society's ideas of need. However, under the existing system, as Cooper notes,

Rationing ... has never been explicitly organized, but has hidden behind each doctor's clinical freedom to act solely in the interests of his patient. Any conflict of interest between patients has been implicitly resolved by the doctor's judgments as to their relative need for care and attention'. [Cooper, 1974, p. 106]

Pricing is an alternative method of rationing by which care is provided to those who value it most highly. Its use as a rationing device would largely (although not entirely) supplant the doctor's role as a rationer. Doctors to a certain extent may lose the power to decide whom they see and when they see them. Another consequence of rationing by price is likely to be the reduction of waiting times (e.g. for an appointment with a doctor, at doctors' surgeries or for admission to hospital). In the absence of money prices, waiting time, it is argued, can act as a price and therefore has a role in rationing care. As demand increases, waiting time may increase (particularly if supply remains unchanged), and as a result some individuals may not demand care. The idea that higher-earned-income groups have a higher opportunity cost of time and therefore find queuing more costly than lower-income groups has been advanced as a reason for preferring non-monetary rationing by waiting time to money price rationing. 'Since time is more equally distributed than money, this rationing device may be thought to be desirable because of equity considerations. . . .' (Nichols *et al.*, 1971). Several arguments have been advanced against this view. Time spent consulting a doctor is likely to mean a loss of pay to the hourly paid worker, whereas this is not generally the case for salaried workers. Further, any discrimination is on the basis of earned income and not on the level of unearned income, which does not affect the opportunity cost of time.[3]

The special role of doctors in the health care market may, however, undermine the advantages claimed for pricing. Feldstein (1974) argues that, because patients lack the technical knowledge to make the necessary decisions, they delegate authority to physicians. This 'agency relationship' develops because of the costs to the patient of acquiring the information that he requires in order to make his own decisions:

> If the agency relation is complete, i.e. if the physician acts solely in the interest of his patient, it would be difficult if not impossible to distinguish the agency relation from the traditional model of independent consumer behavior on the basis of the observed household consumption of hospital services. . . . But the agency relation is not complete. The physician's decisions will generally reflect not only his patient's preferences, but also his own self interest, the pressures from his professional colleagues, a sense of medical ethics and a concern to make good use of hospital resources. [Feldstein, 1974, p. 383]

Evans (1974) argues that the information differential between physician and patient enables the physician to exert direct non-price influence on the demand for his own services, and that, as a result, the primary role of price is not to balance supply and demand, but to determine physicians' incomes.[4]

One argument sometimes made in favour of introducing the wider use of pricing in the NHS is that it would provide additional revenue and thus permit the devotion of a greater share of the nation's resources to health care (see for example British Medical Association, 1977). We do not consider the merits or otherwise of the different potential sources of finance for the NHS in this chapter, but we note that if, as may be argued, the government's allocation of resources among their competing uses is influenced by the preferences of the community as a whole, and not by the way the money is raised, it would be quite rational for them to offset any increased revenue from charges by a reduction in the contributions from other sources.

It is often argued that zero prices cause 'frivolous' or 'trivial' use of health services. Frivolous or trivial use is usually taken to be that which is not 'medically necessary',[5] medical necessity being adjudged by doctors. Doctors are able to refuse to treat cases they regard as frivolous. However, some consultation time is usually required to determine whether a demand is frivolous, and charges for initial visits to GPs (perhaps only nominal charges) are commonly proposed to deter such use. It may be the case however that even nominal charges would deter, in addition to some frivolous use, also some cases of genuine need – in which case the existence of the former might be an acceptable cost of ensuring that the latter is avoided. With zero prices, an individual's valuation of the benefit of treatment *to him* carries little weight (although persistence might eventually obtain consultation and treatment). It is likely that cases which the GP regard as trivial may not be trivial to the patient. Pricing gives an individual greater opportunity to show *his own* belief of the value of treatment and the urgency with which he requires it.

The use of a price mechanism will not necessarily obviate problems of 'over-consumption', since if a price mechanism was used to ration health care it is highly probable, because of the uncertainty characterising one's demand for health care, that there would come into existence a number of insurance schemes, and that these schemes would also reduce the price at the point of contact. If the individual's demand for care is at all responsive to its price, he will alter his desired expenditures on health care because of the existence of insurance. Each individual may be aware that, by consuming more care, simply because insurance has reduced the price to him at the point of contact, he will cause the premium he must pay to rise. However, no individual has any incentive to restrain his consumption because the benefit to him of higher consumption is great compared with the additional cost he will incur since the costs of his actions will be spread over a large number of premium-payers (Pauly, 1971). Such increased usage, resulting from insurance which lowers the price at the point of contact, has been termed 'moral hazard'. Because of the existence of moral hazard most insurance schemes embody co-insurance rates or other devices which ensure that the price at the point of contact is not zero.[6]

The existence of positive prices reduces the 'over-consumption' resulting from moral hazard but involves costs in terms of reduced risk-spreading. Positive prices may also benefit society by deterring some cases where the cost exceeded the value of the treatment – but at the cost of deterring individuals the treatment of whom would have benefited society. These conflicts of objectives can be overcome in part by very similar policies. It has been suggested that one answer to the problem of moral hazard is the introduction of insurance plans that specify particular levels of reimbursement for particular expenses associated with particular conditions (Zeckhauser, 1970; Marshall, 1976). In the case of zero prices the problem of frivolous or trivial demands may be partly overcome by specifying what kind of conditions ought to receive what type and amount of care. Essentially, what is required is to operationalise the concept of need. Obviously, neither more nearly specifying states of nature in insurance contracts nor specifying need is costless or easy.

The difficulties and costs of specifying need, it could be argued, can explain the emphasis on 'equal access' as an objective of health care in the United Kingdom. The very limited role of the price mechanism in the NHS would seem to imply that one aim was to provide care to those whom society thought needed it. This principle can be found as a statement of policy in an oft-quoted passage from the 1944 White Paper on a National Health Service:

> The Government ... want to ensure that in future every man and woman and child can rely on getting ... the best medical and other facilities available; that their getting these shall not depend on whether they can pay for them, or on any other factor irrelevant to ... real need. [Ministry of Health, 1944, p. 5]

However, the government does not define strictly and categorically for doctors those instances where treatment is needed and the decisions are left to the doctors themselves. Possibly as a result of the non-specification of need, the objective frequently upheld as underlying the NHS is that of 'equal access' – that there should be no barriers that discriminate more strongly against one set of people than another. Desires for 'equal access' arguably flow from the concern of one individual for another that we have discussed above. The objective of 'equal access' differs from one explicitly in terms of need in that the former is a simpler and less comprehensive formulation of the latter.

The major reason for limiting the role of prices, therefore, appears to be concern over their deterrent effects. We note that the existing UK system is virtually at one extreme – that characterised by the absence of pricing. An important question to be asked is whether or not society would be better off if we moved away from this position and increased the use of charges on the consumer. Would a system where we charged all those above, and exempted all those below, a certain level of income represent an improvement? Is it desirable to charge a zero price for all treatments, or could we benefit from pricing *some* services above zero, while keeping others 'free'? We cannot answer these questions here, since they depend largely on individuals' valuations of different outcomes, about which we have little information. In the next section we consider some of the evidence available on the empirical issues, in particular on the deterrent effect of prices.

7.3 EVIDENCE

The evidence we shall review in this section tends to be more in terms of assessing the possible *disadvantages* of pricing rather than the advantages. This is because the major advantages claimed for pricing are that it allocates resources more efficiently than a system not using prices and that it permits individuals greater freedom of choice. What constitutes relevant evidence on these issues is not entirely clear, although international comparisons between countries using and not using a price mechanism to allocate health care may be of some help. The evidence upon which this paper concentrates concerns the effects of prices on the demand by consumers for health care. This kind of evidence cannot by its very nature support propositions as to whether pricing is advantageous, but rather permits some consideration of its disadvantageous aspects.

7.3.1   The price elasticity of demand

The own-price elasticity of demand measures the responsiveness of the quantity demanded to changes in the price of the good. If the change in the quantity demanded, resulting from a change in the good's price, is proportionately greater/less than the change in its price, we say that demand is elastic/inelastic. In general we would expect demand to fall as price rises, i.e. we expect the elasticity to be negative. This expectation has tended to be confirmed by the evidence, although there are a number of exceptions. For example, an early study by Feldstein and Severson (1964) found price elasticities largely not significantly different from zero, and when demand was measured in terms of hospital expenditures a positive and significant elasticity (0.43) was found. A number of criticisms can be made of this study, as with virtually all the empirical work we shall review. We shall briefly outline some of these, a fuller discussion being contained in Newhouse and Phelps (1974a). The value of the own-price elasticity tells us the extent to which demand will rise or fall when price changes. In other words, it can tell us the degree to which people are likely to be deterred from demanding health care if the price is increased. Unfortunately, largely as a result of the lack of appropriate data, there is considerable doubt as to the accuracy of many of the estimates of elasticity that have been made. The estimated elasticities have a relatively wide range. The most obvious reason for a variety of estimates is the non-homogeneous nature of the good 'health care' – we would not expect the demand for all services to be similar. One factor that will influence the size of the elasticity will be the existence, or otherwise, of substitutes for the treatment. All the studies that we consider below, unless otherwise stated, are based on US data.

7.3.2   The demand for general hospital services

Rosenthal (1970) presents some evidence on elasticities of demand for short-term general hospital services in New England in 1962. He estimates elasticities for a number of medical and surgical categories which range from −0.24 to −0.70 when length of stay is the measure of quantity demanded, and from −0.30 to −0.97 using post-operative length of stay.[7] His work has been criticised on the grounds that his price variables, cash payment as a percentage of total bill and average daily room charge, do not measure the prices faced by the consumer. Also, the omission of variables from his equations is likely to mean that the elasticities are biased (Fuchs, 1970).

Joseph (1972) estimates price elasticities for twenty-two separate illnesses or conditions. He derives these elasticities by comparing the length of stay of patients with and without insurance. He treats insured patients as if they face a zero money price and the uninsured as if they face some unspecified positive money price. This approach would appear to be unlikely to yield very reliable results. He describes his results according to whether the demand was elastic, inelastic or of the 'wrong sign' (positive) but does not present his estimated equations or sufficient information to enable one to determine whether or not the estimated elasticities are significantly different from zero. He finds the demand to be inelastic for thirteen International Morbidity Code categories, elastic for two and the wrong sign for seven categories. Joseph observed a tendency for third-party payments to affect the length of stay more for the less serious illnesses or conditions; he also noted that patients with the more serious conditions were less sensitive to price. For both the categories for which elastic demands were computed (primary atypical pneumonia and fracture of neck of femur) there were lower-cost alternatives to an extra day in hospital. In other words, patients were most responsive to the price of hospital care when there were good substitutes available for such care. Chiswick (1976) also presents evidence of elastic demand where there are close substitutes available. Using a price variable based on the monthly charge to residents in nursing homes, he estimated an own-price elasticity of demand for nursing home care for the aged of -2.3.

Using 1972 data from thirteen group-family insurance plans in Kentucky, *Freiberg and Scutchfield (1976)* estimate the elasticity of demand for hospital inpatient services. They use out-of-pocket cost (that part of the bill that must be paid by the household) as a measure of price. With admissions per 1000 contracts as the dependent variable, they estimate the price elasticity as -0.299, and with average length of stay as the dependent variable it is -0.069. It seems likely that their results will be biased as a result of their omitting important variables from their analysis. Also, their results are based on a very small sample size. A further problem may be caused by those people who expect to use relatively greater care choosing insurance policies with relatively low co-insurance rates.

Feldstein (1971) pooled cross-section and time series data for individual states from 1958 to 1967. He used an insurance variable which represented the proportion of expenditure on short-term hospital services paid by consumers to convert the average cost per patient-day in short-term general hospitals into a net price facing consumers in each state. Measuring the quantity demanded by a demographically adjusted admission rate, he estimated the elasticity with respect to net price to be equal to -0.626; and measuring demand by demographically adjusted mean stay per admission the elasticity was -0.494. When variables measuring physician and hospital bed availability are introduced, these fall to -0.435 and -0.236, respectively, yielding a price elasticity for hospital days of -0.67.

Davis and Russell (*1972*), using data on forty-eight states for the year 1969, estimated price elasticities of demand for admission to hospital ranging from -0.19 to -0.46 depending on which measure of inpatient price was used. Measuring demand in terms of mean length of stay, the range of elasticities was $+0.35$ to -0.30.[8] Newhouse and Phelps (1974a) argue that the specification of the insurance variable led to inconsistent estimates of the coefficient of the gross price variable in Davis and Russell's study. Their work suggests that including the gross price with an insurance dummy rather than the marginal price in the equation overestimates the price elasticity.[9]

Newhouse and Phelps (*1974b*), using 1963 household survey data, estimate the own-price elasticity of demand for hospital care as -0.10 using ordinary least squares (OLS) and -0.03 using two-stage least squares (2SLS). The price variable that they use, derived by multiplying the gross price by the individual's co-insurance rate, has the advantage of measuring the marginal price faced by the consumer.

7.3.3   The demand for general physicians' services

As can be seen from the above studies, the price elasticities of demand for hospital inpatient care that have been estimated fall in a relatively wide range, although they are generally inelastic. We now turn to estimates of the price elasticities for GP and outpatient visits and for physicians' services in general.

Davis and Russell (*1972*) found that the price elasticity of demand for outpatient visits lay between -0.98 and -1.03. They measured the price of outpatient visits as gross outpatient revenue per outpatient visit. Owing to the absence of data on prices, a number of studies have used a similar procedure to obtain estimates of price (Feldstein and Severson, 1964; Feldstein, 1970; Holtmann and Olsen, 1976).[10]

Newhouse and Phelps (*1974b*) estimate the price elasticity of demand for physician office visits as -0.06 by OLS and -0.02 by 2SLS, and estimate the price elasticity of demand for non-surgical physician visits as -0.10 by OLS and -0.03 by 2SLS (1974a). They argue that OLS estimates are inconsistent away from zero, whereas 2SLS estimates are consistent. Most studies have in fact used OLS to estimate price elasticities. Fuchs and Kramer (1972) use 2SLS to estimate the price elasticity of demand for physician visits from data for thirty-three states in 1966. Using average price, their elasticities fall in the range of -0.104 to -0.356, and using net price (average price net of insurance) in the range of -0.153 to -0.201. As a result of data limitations they are forced to use rather crude measures of price and of quantity demanded.

Feldstein (*1970*) found that the estimated price elasticity of demand for physicians' services with respect to net price (i.e. price net of insurance) was always positive. Brown and Lapan (1972) suggested that this result was caused by Feldstein's choice of price variable. However, when they re-estimated the equation correcting for this, they still obtained positive price elasticities. These and other positive price elasticities occasionally observed may be a product of the special role of doctors in the health care market, referred to in Section 7.2 above. Medical ethics may constrain the doctors' ability to ration demand by price, and professional interests may encourage doctors to keep price at a level that generates excess demand, thus enabling them to be selective about whom they treat. Therefore, the observed prices and quantities may not be points on the demand curve, so that the elasticity estimated would not be a demand elasticity (Feldstein, 1974).

Rosett and Huang (1973) estimate price elasticities of demand for hospitalisation and physicians' services using 1960 household data. They find price elasticities ranging from -0.35 to -1.5. Phelps and Newhouse (1974a) present a number of reasons for believing that these are overestimates of the true elasticity.

In contrast to these relatively large elasticities, *Phelps and Newhouse (1974b)*, in their survey of selected studies, noted much lower elasticities (in absolute terms), e.g. for hospital services -0.14, for ambulatory ancillary services -0.07, for home visits -0.35, for prescription drugs -0.07, for dental care -0.07. One likely explanation for this is that their elasticity estimates were derived for a 0 to 25 per cent range of co-insurance rates, whereas those of Rossett and Huang are estimated for higher rates of co-insurance.

7.3.4   The demand for other health services

Using data for the seven dental regions in the United States for 1956, 1959, 1962, 1965 and 1968, *Feldstein (1973)* estimated the price elasticity of demand for dental visits to be -1.43. Owing to a lack of data the model he estimated was a very simple one.

A very much lower price elasticity was estimated by *Holtmann and Olsen (1976)* using data from a survey of households in New York and Pennsylvania made during 1971–2. They found that the money–price elasticity of demand ranged from -0.032 to -0.187 and that the money–price elasticity tended to be higher (in absolute value) for lower income groups. An interesting feature of their analysis which we consider below was the inclusion of waiting time and travel time. They created their money price variable by dividing the family's total expenditure on dental visits by the number of visits.

Although some research is being carried out on the effects of charges in the NHS, little is yet available upon which to comment. *Lavers (1977)* investigated the demand for prescription drugs in England over the period January 1967 to December 1974. Using monthly data and including variables to measure morbidity, income, seasonal factors, the price of related goods and the price of prescriptions, he estimated a linear and a log linear model. The former yielded an own-price elasticity of demand of -0.06 and the latter, -0.02.[11] Since these elasticities were estimated for all prescriptions, for roughly half of which no payment is made, the price elasticity for prescriptions that have been paid for will be somewhat higher.

The studies reviewed above have in general the common finding that demand is inelastic, though there is little agreement about the degree of inelasticity. In other words, consumers are not highly responsive to changes in the price of care – a 10 per cent rise in price will always cause a less than 10 per cent fall in demand. This implies that charging for health care could be an effective means of raising revenue.

7.3.5 The effects of introducing a pricing system

The above evidence on the elasticities of demand for health care is derived from a wide variety of locations, populations and insurance schemes. It is therefore of interest to examine studies of a more experimental nature, where the effects of the introduction of pricing after an initial situation of free medical care can be seen more clearly. We concentrate here on three North American experiments, there being next to no analysis of pricing in the United Kingdom.

(i) *The Palo Alto experiment.* From December 1965 a comprehensive insurance plan for medical care (the Group Health Plan – GHP) was offered to employees of Stanford University working at least 50 per cent of full time and their dependents. From 1 April 1967, a 25 per cent co-insurance provision was applied: i.e., members had to pay, in addition to their premiums, 25 per cent of the customary charge for any clinic service they used.

(ii) *The Saskatchewan experiment.* From July 1962, compulsory insurance coverage for medical care was introduced for virtually all residents of the province. From April 1968 to August 1971, a co-payment policy was introduced allowing all physicians to charge

$1.50 for office visits;

$2.00 for home, emergency or hospital outpatient visits.

(iii) *California's Medi-Cal Co-payment experiment.* From March 1966, free medical services were available to those persons defined as 'medically needy'.[12] Between 1 January 1972 and 30 June 1973, potential Medi-Cal beneficiaries above certain specified 'wealth' levels were required to pay

$1.00 for each of their first two visits to providers each month;

50¢ for each of their first two prescriptions each month.

(a) The Palo Alto experiment

For the Palo Alto study, Scitovsky and Snyder (1972) considered changes in the number of physician visits per head over the same persons both before and after co-insurance, according to the specialty of the physician (table 7.1). The percentage reduction in visits is substantial, although we cannot be sure that this is entirely due to co-insurance because, although the same people were considered in both 1966 and 1968, certain of their characteristics that might influence the number of visits (such as size of family or income) may have changed. While the extent of changes in characteristics between 1966 and 1968 may have been small, their omission may cause some error in interpretation of results. In addition, we cannot be sure that the decrease in visits was not related to some external factor (e.g. a very mild winter), or chance.

TABLE 7.1

Percentage change in number of physician visits per head, 1966–1968, by field of specialty

General practice	−21.9%
Medical	−21.9%
Surgical	−30.9%
Radiology	−12.6%

Source: Scitovsky and Snyder (1972, table 11).

Those specialties showing small declines in utilisation rates (less than 10 per cent) were dermatology and obstetrics/gynaecology. Those showing large declines (greater than 35 per cent) were allergy, orthopaedics and urology. To consider the question of over-utilisation, a further study of GHP members was carried out. Data were collected on diagnoses of members directly from records, for the two years. The findings – that the number of attended cases of minor complaints[13] declined by 22.5 per cent from 1966 to 1968, compared with a decline in the total number of attended cases of illness of 17.5 per cent – were considered to be 'suggestive rather than conclusive', because of reservations about the accuracy of data.

(b) The Saskatchewan experiment

Beck, in a study of the Saskatchewan experiment, does not unfortunately provide directly comparable data. Services received are grouped broadly (Beck, 1974), and the analysis of data by various medical services has at present been carried out only for the poor.[14] By using regression techniques, Beck standardised for any changes in size of family, age of family head and income to obtain an estimate of the reduction in utilisation that was directly due to co-payment. By comparing this with mean utilisation of services, he estimated percentage reductions in utilisation owing to co-payment (table 7.2).

TABLE 7.2

Percentage change in utilisation of services by the poor (owing to co-payment)

GP services	− 14%
Specialist	− 5%
Home and emergency visits	− 27%
Hospital visits	− 16%
Laboratory services*	− 6%
Major surgery*	− 8%
Minor surgery*	− 13%

Source: Beck (1974, table 3).

* As these were not subject to co-payment, the effects of co-payment were indirect.

(c) The Californian experiment

The Californian experiment interviewed people before and after the introduction of co-payment about their utilisation of medical services in the previous four weeks. Two groups of persons could be distinguished from their sample – those who were subject to co-payment, and those who were not. While we are interested primarily in the change in utilisation among the first group, the second group can serve as a 'control' group, in case factors other than the introduction of co-payment influenced the change in utilisation between the two dates.[15] From table 7.3 it appears that co-payment had little effect on utilisation of medical services. The experiment was designed to examine in detail the effect of co-payment on the receipt of care for 'significant' and 'insignificant' health problems, and health conditions were therefore finely classified. Several hundred symptoms and conditions were perceived by three physicians and categorised into four degrees of seriousness, defined according to the likelihood of (i) death, disability or impairment, and (ii) severe risk of pain, discomfort or depression if the condition were left untreated. The four categories were 'significant', 'intermediate', 'insignificant' and 'indeterminate' (doctors failed to agree).[16]

TABLE 7.3

Changes in the percentage reporting item in past four-week period 1971–2

Type of service	Those subject to co-payment	Those not subject to co-payment
Doctor visits	+0.3%	+0.3%
Visits for injections, X-rays, tests, exams	+1.1%	−0.1%
Prescriptions filled	+2.2%	−0.8%
Dental visit	+2.2%	0
Regular care if pregnant	+0.2%	+3.9%

Source: Brian and Gibbens (1974, p. 31).

Table 7.4 gives the change in percentage of those seeing a doctor for the first illness reported. For significant illnesses, there is no great difference in utilisation change between co-payers and non-co-payers. There is a clear difference between the two groups for both intermediate and insignificant illnesses. Payment of $1.00 for a first visit to a doctor does therefore seem to deter those individuals with 'insignificant' illnesses. To give a particular example, it was found that, after co-payment was in operation, and considering only those individuals belonging to a family deprived of parental support, 26.7 per cent of reported colds resulted in a visit to the doctor in a four-week period by those not co-paying, compared with only 15.2 per cent by those co-paying.

TABLE 7.4

Change in the percentage seeing a doctor for first illness reported
1971–2

Significance of illness	Those subject to co-payment	Those not subject to co-payment
Significant	−0.3%	+1.1%
Intermediate	−12.2%	−2.3%
Insignificant	−4.7%	+3.7%

Source: Brian and Gibbens (1974, from table W–43).

The large difference in utilisation for intermediate illnesses caused by co-payment does seem to give some cause for concern. For those intermediate conditions when a doctor was not seen, co-payment was never specifically mentioned as the reason for not seeing the doctor. However, in 13.9 per cent of these conditions those co-paying named financial reasons, whereas non-co-payers named financial reasons in only 4.5 per cent of cases (Brian and Gibbens, 1974, table W–37).

These results from the Californian study highlight the importance of examining how co-payment affects the structure of GP visits rather than visits in total. While one may not agree exactly with the classification of the illnesses into groups, it is likely that this approach is the more useful. However, the design of the Californian experiment can be criticised. The use of a control group of non-co-payers chosen on the basis of their (lack of) wealth reduces the relevance of comparisons between the groups, as wealth is believed directly to influence utilisation, and any external events or trends may affect each group differently. Multivariate analysis (as used by Beck) applied to those co-paying would have isolated any effect of co-payment on utilisation more directly, while at the same time controlling for income, etc.

Enterline *et al.* (1973) looked at a policy the opposite of those above –

where a 'free' health service replaced a system of direct patient payments for medical care. They found that the proportion of people visiting a physician for common symptoms 'for which medical care would be important' increased from 62 to 73 per cent when prices were reduced to zero. They concluded that Medicare (the free medical care system in Canada) 'may result in some improvements in health'. While the figures may not apply under the reverse policy (of introducing pricing), the evidence does not favour the view that health states are unaffected by pricing.[17]

Pricing is often put forward as a means of reducing the 'frivolous' or 'unnecessary' use of medical services thought prevalent under a system of free medical care. Little evidence is available on this issue. However, Wolfson and Solari (1976) found that under the Ontario Health Insurance Plan (a compulsory universal system with no point-of-use charges) there was no statistically significant evidence of such 'abuse' – patient consultation rates were almost entirely explained by health status measures of the patients. To the extent that there was any abuse at all, it seemed to be generated from the physician side rather than the patient side, caused by the financial incentives confronting physicians under the Ontario fee-per-service system of doctor remuneration.

7.3.6   The effects of pricing on the prevention of illness

 From an economic point of view, there is clearly a trade-off between spending money now on prevention and spending (possibly more) money later on curing those illnesses that might previously have been prevented or restricted. We cannot be certain of the extent by which prevention might be preferable to cure, as this will depend on the costs involved, the preferences for spending now rather than later, and other tastes of individuals.

A priori, having to pay for health care according to services received might be thought to induce an individual to be more concerned about his health status. He might therefore think more carefully about any action that might affect his health (e.g. hang-gliding, cigarette smoking). The individual would then be made more aware that there are costs to other people (in terms of health care resources used) as well as to himself of such activities.

 Also, he might take steps to ensure that illnesses are diagnosed before they become more expensive (to the individual at least) to heal (e.g., going regularly for medical examinations or at first sign of illness). However, pricing might counteract this, so that the net effect of pricing on prevention is uncertain. In Palo Alto, the number of annual physical exams fell by 18.5 per cent after the introduction of a co-insurance rate. In the Californian experiment, which imposed a fixed sum per GP visit and did not charge for inpatient hospital care, the percentage change in the number of physical check-ups per head was an *increase* of 93.4 per cent for those subject to co-payment and an *increase* of 80.4 per cent for those not subject to co-payment. Figures for other preventive services are available only for the Californian experiment and are given in table 7.5.

It is clear that the evidence in California does not suggest that co-payment causes individuals to put off preventive treatment. However, neither does co-payment appear to cause an increase in the use of preventive services, since the control group of non-co-payers also uses more of them. The large increase in prevention services for both groups observed in California suggests, that important factors have been omitted from the investigation. Because of this, and because the control group was chosen on the basis of wealth, we cannot deduce the direction of the net effect of co-payment on utilisation of preventive services in the Californian experiment.

TABLE 7.5

Percentage change in the number of services received per head (in previous six months) 1971–2

Services	Those subject to co-payment	Those not subject to co-payment
Physical check-ups	+ 93.4%	+ 80.4%
Chest X-rays	+ 30.4%	+ 22.6%
Inoculations/vaccinations	+160.7%	+138.2%
Eye exams	+ 91.2%	+ 57.7%
Pap smears	− 5.4%	− 3.3%

Source: Calculated from Brian and Gibbens (1974, table W–16).

Evidence from two US states has suggested that the greater the price of medical care facing the individual, the less likely he is to seek physical exams (Salkever, 1976), thus supporting the findings from Palo Alto. However, no proper account was taken of the possible interactions involved when GP and hospital payments are not *both* involved, and when GP and hospital visits may act as substitutes. Alternatively, pricing may reduce 'medically necessary' visits to GPs and result later in (possibly more costly) visits to a hospital when the illness has become more serious. For example, in a study of the effects of a utilisation fee imposed for GP visits but not for hospitalisation, it was found that the reduction in GP visits 'was immediately accompanied by a partially offsetting increase in the incidence of hospital visits ... and by a significant increase in minor surgery' (Straight, 1962, as quoted in Hall, 1966, p. 257). A similar dichotomy of payments also occurred in the Californian experiment, and it was noticed that the hospitalisation rate for those subject to co-payment increased relative to those not co-paying after charges were introduced for GP visits (Roemer *et al.*, 1975).

From the evidence so far available, we cannot be certain whether the increased use of hospitals was due to a reduction of medical care at the GP level, leading to illnesses becoming more developed and serious before contact is made with the health system, or whether hospital visits were used as a substitute for GP visits. These possible long-term effects of prices are likely to be as important as the short-term effects, and should not be ignored when evidence on pricing is presented.

7.3.7 An indirect approach to examining the demand for care

Because the analysis of pricing so far carried out has often been of too general a nature to examine directly the effects of pricing on needed and frivolous health care use, a more indirect approach must be used for this. If, for example, it could be argued that the need for medical care strikes at random between income groups, say, then if an objective of giving care according to need was accomplished, we would not expect to find income important in determining medical service utilisation. Similarly, if lower income groups were thought to need more care than higher income groups, we would not expect to find that income causes significantly greater utilisation. By examining the importance of income in determining utilisation, we cannot however ever show that care is given according to need, even if we specify how 'need' varies with income (if at all), because such comparisons are relative rather than absolute.

If one considers first those studies that have examined cases where there are no charges facing the individual, then there is increasing evidence that income is still an important factor in determining the use made of health services – those with higher incomes making greater use.[18] This would seem to indicate that health care is received on some basis other than severity of illness, particularly as many studies have indicated that wealthier families seem less prone to illness than other families. For example, the National Center for Health Statistics (1974) showed that the number of restricted activity days per person experienced by low-income families was almost three times greater than the number experienced by high-income families.[19,20]

If we recall the special role of doctors, it would seem advantageous to distinguish between patient-initiated and doctor-initiated visits. However, the difference between these two types of visit is not always clear-cut, and a useful substitute may be to classify the initial contact with the GP separately from subsequent revisits. Richardson (1970) made this distinction and found evidence to suggest that when non-serious conditions (as defined by physicians) are considered, and when the consumer faces zero-prices, then income plays a minor role (at the most) for initial visits, but a more important one for revisits. For serious conditions, 'the differences between poor and non-poor ... are small or non-existent in terms of both visits and revisits' (p. 141). Hershey et al. (1975) also point out the importance of distinguishing between types of visit, but unfortunately few other studies categorise GP visits in this manner.

If, when individuals are faced with zero charges, those with higher incomes (possibly lower 'need') use health services more than those with lower incomes (possibly higher 'need'), then any effect of pricing on the allocation of care according to need can be analysed in terms of the extent by which this difference in usage between high- and low-income groups is made greater.

The Palo Alto experiment classified participants according to one of three occupational groups (at Stanford University), in the absence of data on family income. These were faculty staff (assumed highest paid here), other professional staff, and non-professional staff (assumed lowest paid). We might expect that the highest paid members were least affected by the introduction of co-insurance, so that their utilisation of medical services changed the least. In their study of the experiment, Scitovsky and Snyder (1972) examined the use made of medical services by the same persons both before and after the introduction of co-insurance and deduced from table 7.6 that 'there is some evidence that the lowest socio-economic group, the non-professionals, responded more than the two other occupational categories ... and reduced its use of physician services more' (p. 7). This evidence appears weak, particularly for males, and the group 'Other professional' gives inconsistent results. Because of the special role of doctors, it may be that once the GP has been contacted individuals will be less deterred by price if the GP suggests that the patient revisit him. Thus, as opposed to examining total GP visits, we might examine the number of initial GP visits. However, data on this are unavailable, and one alternative might be to examine the percentage of members who do not see a GP in a year (table 7.7). The evidence does show

TABLE 7.6

Percentage change in number of physician visits per head, 1966–8 (adjusted for age variations between the two dates)

	Total	Male	Female
Faculty	−24.7%	−20.2%	−28.1%
Other professional	−23.5%	−26.7%	−21.0%
Non-professional	−27.4%	−20.2%	−32.4%

Source: Scitovsky and Snyder (1972, table 5).

a much larger difference between income groups after the introduction of co-insurance as compared with table 7.6, particularly for male non-professional members, for whom the proportion with no visits doubled. One of the problems of using the Scitovsky and Snyder method of analysis is that, although the same people were examined both before and after co-insurance, there may be significant differences between income groups in terms of characteristics that might influence physician visits (e.g. age, location of home and size of family). For example, it may be that faculty families generally happen to live further away from clinics than non-professional families, so that the charge for visits is less important to them (being a smaller percentage of total costs when travel costs are included). This deficiency was put right by Phelps and Newhouse (1972), who for the same experiment used multiple regression analysis, so that the effects of age, distance from clinic and family size can be held constant when utilisation by occupation groups is considered. Phelps and Newhouse found that the decrease in the number of physician visits was *not* related to an individual being in any of the three occupation groups (Phelps and Newhouse, 1972, table B). Neither was the decrease in the total number of ancillary services (i.e. X-rays, physical therapy, etc.) used so related.

TABLE 7.7

Percentage of GHP members with no physician visits, 1966 and 1968

	Males 1966	1968	Females 1966	1968
Faculty	12.4%	16.8%	10.3%	13.3%
Other professional	17.7%	25.4%	12.3%	18.9%
Non-professional	15.0%	30.1%	13.9%	21.7%

Source: Scitovsky and Snyder (1972, table 9).

It is worth noting here that the decrease in demand (in terms of physician visits and use of ancillary services) was generally not significantly related to age or family size. However, the change in demand was significantly related to an individual's sex and relationship to the subscriber – adult female dependents of the subscriber being particularly affected by co-insurance. Co-insurance does therefore seem to have some differential impact in this respect.

The authors point out two shortcomings of their study which leave some effects of co-insurance unexamined. Firstly, some families left the GHP scheme after the introduction of co-insurance and were thus excluded from the study. Those leaving the scheme were likely to be those who decided to join a private insurance scheme, which they expected to be less expensive, or who expected to use medical services on a scale small enough to justify paying fully for each service as it was obtained. Many studies have shown that wealthier families are less prone to illness than other families, and it is possible therefore that those who left the GHP scheme after the introduction of co-insurance were those families with relatively greater wealth. If alternative health schemes are available, then it may be that the co-insurance scheme is imposed mainly on the poorer members of the community.

Secondly, some families did not purchase all their requirements from GHP. Such action is likely to occur because of convenience, time and travel costs. We cannot say for certain whether these families have particular characteristics, although it may be that they consist of those who value time relatively highly. It is possible therefore that an individual paid by the hour makes less use of GHP than an identical individual paid by the month even though they were both members of the scheme.

One further problem noted previously, which was not explicitly mentioned in either of the two studies of the GHP experiment, was that, although the same families were considered in both 1966 and 1968, some of their characteristics influencing their propensity to visit a physician may have changed (e.g. size of family). Beck (1976) managed to overcome some of these problems in his study of the Saskatchewan experiment by using cross-section random samples for the years 1963–71 (co-payment was introduced in 1968) and pooling the data. Data on income were available, and Beck used multiple regression techniques to ascertain their significance in determining the quantity of 'services' received per family, while standardising for differences in size of family, age of family head, etc. Rather than look at whether the *change* in utilisation was affected by income (the approach used by Phelps and Newhouse), Beck examined directly whether the effect of income on the quantity of services received differed once co-payment was introduced. Thus, if the importance of income in determining services received actually increased after the introduction of co-payment, inequalities between income groups over the utilisation of services would be made worse. However, Beck found that there was no evidence to support this (Beck, 1976, table 2). It is interesting to note that in an earlier study (Beck, 1971) of the same experiment, Beck estimated that the effect of co-payment (*per se*) caused an 18 per cent reduction in the use of physicians' services by the poor by the first year of operation but only a 6–7 per cent reduction for the insured population as a whole. However, although the difference in percentage terms is large, it may not be so in absolute terms (because the poor generally use fewer services). In addition, the method of estimating these percentages was not very sophisticated, no indication of their accuracy was given, and it was based on a smaller sample than his 1976 study; so we should not put too much emphasis on this possible conflicting evidence.

Such evidence as we have seen on the effects of co-insurance (or co-payment) on different income groups is conflicting, but would tend to support the hypothesis that, of those remaining under an insurance scheme if co-insurance were introduced, no particular income group would be affected more than any other in the use of medical services. However, there will be a redistributive effect, because these services now have to be paid for at the point of contact, and even if all income groups spent the same amount on health care, the percentage of income devoted to this would be higher for the low-income groups than for high-income groups (ignoring any effects of taxation changes that might occur if the revenue raised from pricing health care were substantial).

Payment for medical care according to the level of income is another possible method of co-insurance or co-payment. Scitovsky and Snyder thought that a 25 per cent co-insurance rate applying to all physician services 'might be suitable for families in the middle to upper income groups. For lower-income families, it may impose too much of a financial barrier (Scitovsky and Snyder, 1972, p. 17). Such reasoning might point to a health system where the poor obtain free medical care but those better off are faced with charges. This may be one basis for the US Medicaid–Medicare system. Although this system seems to have some redistributive effect in giving the poor more medical care (see table 7.8), it is still open to question whether the amount of redistribution was 'enough'.[21]

TABLE 7.8

Number of physician contacts per year in the United States

Income p.a.	1963–4 (before Medicaid–Medicare)	1971 (after Medicaid–Medicare)
< $3,000	4.3	6.0
> $15,000	5.8	5.1

Source: National Center for Health Statistics (1975), quoted in Aday (1976, p. 218).

7.3.8   Time-costs as a price of treatment

As stressed in Section 7.2, the absence of charges does not mean that individuals demanding health care incur no costs. In recent empirical work on the demand for health care, economists have started to examine the importance of patients' time as a cost of treatment.

In a study of the demand for 'free' medical services in New York City, Acton (1975) used the distance from the consumer's residence to the out-patient department as a proxy for the time-cost to the consumer of obtaining treatment. He found that the distance to the outpatient department functioned as a price in determining demand. He found an elasticity of −0.14. He noted that the elasticity with respect to travel time is likely to be 'greater [in absolute value] than −0.14 because people travelling further will tend to take a more rapid form of transportation'. Some indirect support for this is contained in an earlier study, where it was found that the own-price elasticity of demand for public ambulatory care with respect to self-reported travel time ranges from −0.6 to −1.0. The travel-time price elasticity for visits to the offices of private physicians ranged from −0.25

to −0.337. This lower (in absolute terms) time price elasticity of demand for private care was also found when the waiting-time price elasticity was considered, −0.05 for private care compared with −0.12 for 'free' public care (Acton, 1973). In addition, Acton (1975) found that persons with higher earned income (and therefore possibly higher opportunity cost of time) were more likely to use the private sector which is relatively less time-intensive than the public sector.

Holtmann and Olsen (1976), in their study of the demand for dental visits, included in their analysis an estimated money price and a number of variables relating to household characteristics (such as income, number of children, the number of members in the household who were afraid of the dentist). They also had variables representing the time spent waiting at the dentist's surgery per visit and the travelling time involved in the journey from their home to the surgery. They found that the waiting-time price elasticity ranged from −0.054 to −0.255. A similarly low price elasticity was estimated for travel time (−0.121), although their travel time results were less statistically significant (i.e. it is less clear that the result is not due to chance). A further result was that the lowest income class appeared to be the most sensitive to waiting time.

Simon and Smith (1973) examine the effect of distance on utilisation of health services. They consider the number of visits made by students to a 'free' university clinic before and after a change in its location. Using their data Phelps and Newhouse (1974b) estimate the travel-time price elasticity to lie between −0.27 and −0.49.

Phelps and Newhouse (1974a) find that co-insurance affects the demand for services and that the impact of co-insurance varies across medical services in a systematic fashion depending upon the time price of the service. More specifically,

services with a relatively high time price, especially physician office visits, exhibit relatively low coverage (or price) elasticities and relatively high time price elasticities ... services with a relatively high money price such as home visits, show considerably higher own-price elasticities.... Money price elasticities appear to fall with co-insurance rates. [pp. 340–1].

One of the implications of these results for the NHS that can be suggested tentatively is that the money price elasticity of demand would be relatively low for visits to GPs' surgeries if a small payment were instituted (i.e., the number of visits to surgeries would not fall by very much). As the payment rose as a proportion of the total price (i.e. including time-costs) we would expect money price elasticity to increase.

Some further evidence on the role of time-costs is presented by Phelps and Newhouse (1972). They note that the female dependents of the subscribers to the insurance plan that they were studying (many of whom were not in the labour force) made on average 1.66 more visits per year than female subscribers (who were in the labour force). On the assumption that time-cost is higher on the average for female subscribers than for female dependents, this statistically significant difference is evidence on the importance of time-costs in influencing the demand for medical services. Phelps and Newhouse (1974a) note that, after a 25 per cent co-insurance rate was introduced, expenditures on home visits decreased much more than on office visits. The estimated money price elasticities of demand for home visits and office visits were -0.37 and -0.14 respectively. They argue that this difference in the observed money price elasticities is a result of the nearly zero time price of home visits and the substantial time price associated with office visits.

7.4   CONCLUSIONS

Our discussion in Section 7.2, while suggesting a possible rationale for the absence of charges in the NHS – namely that an individual's health is of concern to other people as well as himself – did indicate that universal zero-pricing was not necessarily the only, or the 'best' response to this problem. Whether or not it should be, the preferred policy depends largely on the extent to which charges deter consumption, who is deterred and the value that society places on ensuring that these people do receive treatment. In Section 7.3 we presented evidence on the extent to which charges reduce demand and on who is deterred. At present, we have no information on the value society puts upon any individual's consumption of health care and the extent to which this valuation depends on characteristics of the individual (such as age or income) and on their particular medical condition. Until we obtain information on these matters, it is impossible to say whether society would benefit or suffer from a shift from universal zero-pricing to some form of differential pricing of health care.

NOTES

1. In addition to the other contributors the authors would like to thank Professor J. Wiseman for his comments on an earlier draft of this paper.
2. This concept of need is more restricted than that considered by Culyer (Chapter 2), the major difference being that we are concerned with the costs as well as the potential benefits of treatment.
3. This and other arguments are discussed in Culyer and Cullis (1976).
4. In this chapter we examine evidence on the effect of prices on the consumers of health care. We do not consider how producers (largely doctors) may be influenced by the use of a price mechanism.
5. A more useful concept of frivolous use might be the use of health services that imposes total costs greater than the value to society of such usage.
6. Co-insurance is a form of insurance where the consumer pays C per cent and the insurer pays $(100-C)$ per cent of all expenses. C is known as the co-insurance rate. Other devices are co-payment and deductibles. Co-payment is distinguished from co-insurance by being a fixed sum to be paid for a particular service rather than a

percentage of the price. A deductible specifies the amount that a consumer must pay before the insurance becomes effective.

7. An own-price elasticity of -0.30 implies that when the price of the good or service increases by 10 per cent, the quantity demanded will fall by 3 per cent.

8. The positive elasticity (0.35) was not significantly different from zero. One feature of this study was the inclusion of the price of possible substitutes – in this case of inpatient care, the outpatient price and for outpatient care, the inpatient price. In the outpatient visits and admissions equations these variables were positive and significant, suggesting that their omission would bias the results. Yett *et al.* (1974), also using cross-section state data, found that the cross-price variables were positive. They estimated an own-price elasticity of demand for inpatient care of -0.31.

9. Their estimate of the price elasticity in a hospital length of stay equation falls from -0.55 to -0.29 and for non-surgical physician visits from -0.09 to -0.03, when the equation is specified 'correctly'.

10. The problems associated with measuring price in this way are fully discussed by Newhouse and Phelps (1974a).

11. A similarly low elasticity (-0.07) was estimated by a different method for an earlier period using annual data (1955–69), by Phelps and Newhouse (1974b). In their model they convert the price into a co-insurance rate and do not consider morbidity, income or the price of related goods.

12. Those services freely available in fact depended on whether one was classed in Group I or Group II, but both included free physicians' services, hospital and nursing home care, laboratory services, radiology and prescription drugs.

13. Minor complaints included conditions such as warts, headaches, colds and hay-fever.

14. Roughly, those who spend at least 70 per cent of their income on food, clothing and shelter.

15. Although ideally the control group should be chosen randomly from the total population to be sampled, this was not thought desirable because it would 'impose copayment on beneficiaries whose only resources came from their monthly welfare benefit grant' (Brian and Gibbens, 1974, p. 13). The two groups therefore differed in terms of wealth.

16. Examples of symptoms/conditions in each category are: (i) significant – toxic effects of venom, acute gonococcal infection of the genito-urinary tract, diabetes mellitus, senile dementia, acute appendicitis; (ii) intermediate – peptic ulcer, hepatitis, chronic cystitis of the breast, backache; (iii) insignificant – common cold, loss of appetite, persistent cough, headache; (iv) indeterminate – sore throat, runny nose. The classifications used can be found in full in Brian and Gibbens (1974, Appendix W, pp. 105–48).

17. One of the few studies looking at the effects of the NHS in Britain (Stewart and Enterline, 1961) was unable to show whether 'the increases in physician utilization apparently resulting from the NHS improved the health of the adult population' (p. 1194).

18. For example, see Beck (1973); Beck and Horne (1976); Kovner *et al.* (1969); Le Grand (1976); Manga (1976); Nyman and Kalimo (1973); and Salkever (1975); but see Enterline *et al.* (1973) and Rein (1969) for possible conflicting evidence.

19. See also Rabin and Schach (1975).

20. Although it is probably a commonly held view that those who are sickest need the most care and thus that the less wealthy should make greater use of the health services than those with more income, other factors might also be thought important. For example, incomes might be taken as measures of a person's contribution to production, and society might therefore value the health of those with higher incomes more than those with lower incomes. If this was the case, those with high incomes would need (according to our definition) more health services than those with low incomes. (As a provocative example, one might consider how one values the health of a Cabinet minister, a car assembly line worker and an old age pensioner.) Further discussion of medical and non-medical factors that might be important in determining priority for use of health services is given in Culyer and Cullis (1976).

21. For discussions on the differences in use of medical services between Medicaid–Medicare recipients and others, when some account is taken of health status, see Aday (1976); Bice *et al.* (1972); Hershey *et al.* (1975); Montiero (1973); Olendzki (1974); Rabin *et al.* (1974); Rabin and Schach (1975); and Taylor *et al.* (1975).

REFERENCES

Acton, J. P. (1973) *Demand for Health Care among the Urban Poor with Special Emphasis on the Role of Time* Memorandum R-1151-OEO/NYC, Santa Monica, California, Rand Corporation.

Acton, J. P. (1975) 'Nonmonetary Factors in the Demand for Medical Services: Some Empirical Evidence' *Journal of Political Economy*, vol. 83, no. 3, pp. 595–614.

Aday, L. A. (1976) 'The Impact of Health Policy on Access to Medical Care' *The Millbank Memorial Fund Quarterly* vol. 54, no. 2, pp. 215–33.

Beck, R. G. (1971) 'Analysis of the Demand for Physicians' Services in Saskatchewan' unpublished doctoral dissertation, University of Alberta.

Beck, R. G. (1973) 'Economic Class and Access to Physician Services under Public Medical Care Insurance' *International Journal of Health Services* vol. 3, no. 3, pp. 341–55.

Beck, R. G. (1974) 'The Effects of Copayment on the Poor' *Journal of Human Resources* vol. 9, no. 1, pp. 129–42.

Beck, R. G. (1976) 'Some Dynamic Effects of Copayment on Utilization of Medical Services in Saskatchewan' in Fraser (1976).

Beck, R. G. and Horne, J. M. (1976) 'Economic Class and Risk Avoidance: Experience under Public Medical Care Insurance' *Journal of Risk and Insurance* vol. 43, no. 1, pp. 73–86.

Bice, T. W. Eichhorn, R. L. and Fox, P. D. (1972) 'Socioeconomic Status and Use of Physician Services: a Reconsideration' *Medical Care* vol. 10, no. 3, pp. 261–71.

Brian, E. W. and Gibbens, S. F. (1974) 'California's Medi-Cal Copayment Experiment' *Medical Care* vol. 12, no. 12, supplement.

British Medical Association (1977) 'Royal Commission on the National Health Service – Report of Council to Special Representative Meeting, London, 9 March 1977' *British Medical Journal* 29 January 1977, pp. 299–334.

Brown, D. M. and Lapan, H. E. (1972) 'The Rising Price of Physicians' Services: a Comment' *Review of Economics and Statistics* vol. 54, no. 1, pp. 101–4.

Chiswick, B. R. (1976) 'The Demand for Nursing Home Care: an Analysis of the Substitution Between Institutional and Non-Institutional Care' *Journal of Human Resources* vol. 11, no. 3, pp. 295–316.

Cooper, M. H. (1974) 'Economics of Need: the Experience of the British Health Service' in Perlman (1974).

Culyer, A. J. (1976) *Need and the National Health Service: Economics and Social Choice* London, Martin Robertson.

Culyer, A. J. and Cullis, J. G. (1976) 'Some Economics of Hospital Waiting Lists in the NHS' *Journal of Social Policy* vol. 15, part 3, pp. 239–64.

Davis, K. and Russell, L. B. (1972) 'The Substitution of Hospital Outpatient Care for Inpatient Care' *Review of Economics and Statistics* vol. 54, no. 2, pp. 109–20.

Enterline, P. E., Salter, V., McDonald, A. D. and McDonald, J. C. (1973) 'The Distribution of Medical Services Before and After "Free" Medical Care – the Quebec Experience' *New England Journal of Medicine* vol. 289, part 22, pp. 1174–8.

Evans, R. G. (1974) 'Supplier-Induced Demand' in Perlman (1974).

Feldstein, M. S. (1970) 'The Rising Price of Physicians' Services' *Review of Economics and Statistics* vol. 52, no. 2, pp. 121–33.

Feldstein, M. S. (1971) 'Hospital Cost Inflation: a Study of Non-Profit Price Dynamics' *American Economic Review* vol. 61, no. 5, pp. 853–72.

Feldstein, M. S. (1974) 'Econometric Studies of Health Economics' in Intriligator and Kendrick (1974).

Feldstein, P. J. (1973) *Financing Dental Care: An Economic Analysis* Lexington, Toronto and London, Lexington Books, D. C. Heath & Co.

Feldstein, P. J. and Severson, R. (1964) 'The Demand for Medical Care' in American Medical Association, *Report of the Commission on the Cost of Medical Care* Chicago, American Hospital Association.

Fraser, R. D. (ed.) (1976) *Health Economics Symposium, Proceedings of the First Canadian*

Conference, Industrial Relations Centre, Queen's University, Kingston.

Freiberg, L. and Scutchfield, F. D. (1976) 'Insurance and the Demand for Hospital Care: an Examination of Moral Hazard' *Inquiry* vol. 13, no. 1, pp. 54–60.

Fuchs, V. R. (1970) 'Comment' in Klarman (1970).

Fuchs, V. R. and Kramer, M. J. (1972) *Determinants of Expenditures for Physicians' Services in the United States 1948–1968* Washington, DC, US Government Printing Office.

Hall, C. B. (1966) 'Deductibles in Health Insurance – an Evaluation' *Journal of Risk and Insurance* vol. 33, pp. 253–63.

Hershey, J. C., Luft, H. S. and Gianaris, J. M. (1975) 'Making Sense out of Utilization Data' *Medical Care* vol. 13, no. 10, pp. 838–54.

Holtmann, A. G. and Olsen, E. O. (1976) 'The Demand for Dental Care: A Study of Consumption and Household Production' *Journal of Human Resources* vol. 11, no. 4, pp. 546–60.

Intriligator, M. D. and Kendrick, D. A. (eds) (1974) *Frontiers of Quantitative Economics*, Volume II, Amsterdam and Oxford, North-Holland Publishing Co.

Joseph, H. (1972) 'Hospital Insurance and Moral Hazard' *Journal of Human Resources* vol. 7, no. 2, pp. 152–61.

Klarman, H. E. (ed.) (1970) *Empirical Studies in Health Economics* Baltimore and London, Johns Hopkins Press.

Kovner, J. W., Browne, L. B. and Kisch, A. I. (1969) 'Income and the Use of Outpatient Medical Care by the Insured' *Inquiry* vol. 6, no. 2, pp. 27–34.

Lavers, R. J. (1977) 'A Demand Model for Prescriptions', unpublished paper, Institute of Social and Economic Research, University of York.

Le Grand, J. (1976) 'The Distribution of Public Expenditure: the Case of Health Care' (mimeograph), University of Sussex, Economics Paper series 76/16.

Manga, P. (1976) 'A Benefit Incidence Analysis of the Public Medical and Hospital Insurance Programs in Ontario' unpublished PhD thesis, University of Toronto.

Marshall, J. M. (1976) 'Moral Hazard' *American Economic Review* vol. 66, no. 5, pp. 880–90.

Ministry of Health (1944) *White Paper on a National Health Service* London, HMSO.

Montiero, L. A. (1973) 'Expense is No Object – Income and Physician Visits Reconsidered' *Journal of Health and Social Behavior* vol. 14, no. 2, pp. 99–115.

National Center for Health Statistics (1974) 'Disability Days: United States, 1971' Series 10, No. 90.

National Center for Health Statistics (1975) 'Physician Visits – Volume and Interval Since Last Visit: United States, 1971' Series 10, No. 97.

Newhouse, J. P. and Phelps, C. E. (1974a) *On Having Your Cake and Eating it Too: Econometric Problems in Estimating the Demand for Health Services*, Memorandum R-1149-NC, Santa Monica, California, Rand Corporation.

Newhouse, J. P. and Phelps, C. E. (1974b) 'Price and Income Elasticities for Medical Care Services' in Perlman (1974).

Nichols, D., Smolensky, E. and Tideman, T. N. (1971) 'Discrimination by Waiting Time in Merit Goods' *American Economic Review* vol. 61, no. 2, part 1, pp. 312–23.

Nyman, K. and Kalimo, E. (1973) 'Physicians' Services in Finland' *Social Science and Medicine* vol. 7, no. 7, pp. 541–53.

Olendzki, M. C. (1974) 'Medicaid Benefits Mainly the Younger and Less Sick' *Medical Care* vol. 12, no. 2, pp. 163–72.

Pauly, M. V. (1971) *Medical Care at Public Expense – A Study in Applied Welfare Economics* New York and London, Praeger.

Perlman, Mark (ed.) (1974) *The Economics of Health and Medical Care* proceedings of a conference held by the International Economic Association at Tokyo. London, Macmillan.

Phelps, C. E. and Newhouse, J. P. (1972) 'Effect of Coinsurance: a Multivariate Analysis' *Social Security Bulletin* vol. 35, no. 6, pp. 20–44.

Phelps, C. E. and Newhouse, J. P. (1974a) 'Coinsurance, the Price of Time, and the Demand for Medical Services' *Review of Economics and Statistics* vol. 56, no. 3, pp. 334–43.

Phelps, C. E. and Newhouse, J. P. (1974b) *Coinsurance and the Demand for Medical Services* Memorandum R-964-1-OEO/NC. Santa Monica, California, Rand Corporation.

Rabin, D. L., Bice, T. W. and Starfield, B. (1974) 'Use of Health Services by Baltimore Medicaid Recipients' *Medical Care* vol. 12, no. 7, pp. 561–70.

Rabin, D. L. and Schach, E. (1975) 'Medicaid, Morbidity and Physician Use' *Medical Care* vol. 13, no. 1, pp. 68–78.

Rein, M. (1969) 'Social Class and the Utilization of Medical Care Services' *Hospitals* vol. 43, no. 13, pp. 43–54.

Richardson, W. C. (1970) 'Measuring the Urban Poor's Use of Physicians' Services in Response to Illness Episodes' *Medical Care* vol. 8, no. 2, pp. 132–42.

Roemer, M. I., Hopkins, C. E., Carr, L. and Gartside, F. (1975) 'Copayments for Ambulatory Care: Penny-Wise and Pound Foolish' *Medical Care* vol. 13, no. 6, pp. 457–66.

Rosenthal, G. (1970) 'Demand for Short-Term General Hospital Services' in Klarman (1970).

Rosett, R. N. and Huang, L. (1973) 'The Effect of Health Insurance on the Demand for Medical Care' *Journal of Political Economy* vol. 81, no. 2, part 1, pp. 281–305.

Salkever, D. S. (1975) 'Economic Class and Differential Access to Care: Comparisons among Health Care Systems' *International Journal of Health Services* vol. 5, no. 3, pp. 373–95.

Salkever, D. S. (1976) 'Accessibility and the Demand for Preventive Care' *Social Science and Medicine* vol. 10, no. 9/10, pp. 469–75.

Scitovsky, A. A. and Snyder, N. M. (1972) 'Effect of Coinsurance on Use of Physician Services' *Social Security Bulletin* vol. 35, no. 6, pp. 3–19.

Simon, J. L. and Smith, D. B. (1973) 'Change in Location of a Student Health Service; a Quasiexperimental Evaluation of the Effects of Distance on Utilization' *Medical Care* vol. 11, no. 1, pp. 59–67.

Stewart, W. H. and Enterline, P. E. (1961) 'Effects of the National Health Service on Physician Utilization and Health in England and Wales' *New England Journal of Medicine* vol. 265, no. 24, pp. 1187–94.

Straight, Byron W. (1962) 'Reducing the Incidence of Office and Home Visits in a Medical Service Plan by Use of Coinsurance Charges' *Proceedings Conference of Actuaries in Private Practice* vol. 11.

Taylor, D. G., Aday, L. A. and Anderson, R. (1975) 'A Social Indicator of Access to Medical Care' *Journal of Health and Social Behavior* vol. 16, no. 1, pp. 39–49.

Wolfson, A. D. and Solari, A. J. (1976) *Research Report on the Results of the Patient Utilisation Study* unpublished report for the Ontario Ministry of Health.

Yett, D. E., Drabeck, L., Intriligator, M. D. and Kimbell, L. J. (1974) 'Economic Forecasts of Health Services and Health Manpower' in Perlman (1974).

Zeckhauser, R. (1970) 'Medical Insurance: a Case Study of the Trade-Off between Risk Spreading and Appropriate Incentives' *Journal of Economic Theory* vol. 2, no. 1, pp. 10–26.

8. Financing Medical Education – Interrelationships Between Medical School and Teaching Hospital Expenditure

A. J. Culyer and M. F. Drummond[1]

8.1 INTRODUCTION

Medical education differs from many other types of university education in that it involves a mandatory period of practical training in NHS hospitals outside the university's medical school. It has long been recognised that these practical phases of training in teaching hospitals are likely to cause extra expenditure in the NHS. Indeed the average cost (per inpatient case) of teaching hospitals is consistently higher than that of broadly comparable non-teaching hospitals. In a recent study, Culyer *et al.* (1976a) estimate the costs attributable to student presence at £3557 per student per annum (1970 prices). This is at least as high as the universities' unit costs (per student per annum) for clinical medicine (University Grants Committee (UGC), 1975).

The common funding of medical education by both DES (via UGC) and DHSS (via the NHS) raises two general issues.

(i) What should the relative financial contributions of education and health sectors be?
(ii) Can one make sensible comparisons of the relative cost of teaching hospitals or medical schools without consideration of expenditure patterns in *both* sectors?

In tackling the first, one might argue that if the hospital costs attributable to student presence truly represent the cost of education, then it seems natural that the government department explicitly providing funds for education should fund it. However, there is an element of 'jointness' or of inseparability in the teaching and treating functions of the teaching hospital that makes the precise estimation of the true total costs of practical education difficult. For instance, there is always the possibility that some of the costs attributed to student presence arise not merely from the process of teaching, but from a difference in treatment mode or 'style' that would persist even if the students were removed. Also, one has no knowledge of the extent to which the presence of students in the teaching hospital adds to, or detracts from, the value of the treatments provided.[2] Therefore, the net cost of teaching to the NHS could be larger or smaller than the figure estimated. (For a fuller discussion of these points see Culyer et al., 1976b.) Finally, it could be argued that in any case the question of relative funding is of relevance only to those whose budgets are affected. From the community's point of view, medical education and the resulting change in the stock of human capital is either worth having or it is not, irrespective of which government budget provides the funds. What is important is that all the costs and benefits from engaging in medical education are identified and compared with those for other public and private sector projects. In this respect, the estimation of the NHS costs associated with teaching medical students is a step forward.

It is to the second general issue that this paper is directed. The issue of cost comparisons is of interest to administrators in both health and education sectors since, in the absence of a reliable indicator of efficiency, cost comparisons are important in the monitoring of institutional performance.[3] Studies undertaken in both fields in the United Kingdom (e.g. Feldstein, 1967, and Culyer et al., 1976a,b on hospital costs; Verry and Layard, 1975, on university costs) suggest that more reliable cost comparisons can be made by standardisation for the different 'product mix' of institutions. Therefore, given the close links between teaching hospitals and medical schools, there would appear to be an a priori case for further standardisation (say) for expenditure patterns in the medical school when attempting to make cost comparisons between teaching hospitals.

Closer examination of teaching hospital and medical school operation reveals a number of aspects of the interrelationship between expenditure patterns in the two sectors. For example, laboratory services are often shared. Replies to a UGC questionnaire (UGC, 1971) showed that the shared service is sometimes operated by one hospital, sometimes by the medical school, and sometimes by both jointly. Different agreements regarding the relative financial contributions by hospital and medical school exist in each case. Another well-known joint arrangement stems from the dual function of some medical staff. Many university staff hold honorary NHS posts and carry out NHS service work. In return, some NHS staff carry out clinical teaching. A further interrelationship may arise from carrying out research in the medical school. Although most research activity is financed from specific grants, there is the possibility that such activity may necessitate expenditure in the NHS sector.

The validity of cost comparisons between teaching hospitals has acquired a new importance following the report of the DHSS Resource Allocation Working Party (RAWP) (DHSS, 1976). Under the proposed arrangements, teaching hospitals will be funded only up to the level of 75 per cent of the median excess cost of teaching hospitals over a comparative sample of non-teaching hospitals. Application of this allowance (the Service Increment for Teaching, SIFT) on a per student basis to all teaching hospitals leaves the London hospitals comparatively short of funds, since they have the largest residual costs not covered by SIFT (DHSS, 1976). While there are a number of known influences on hospital cost in the metropolis, e.g. the London weighting added to staff salaries, a further relevant factor is the difference observed in the UGC provision to medical schools. The unit cost (per student) in 1973–4 (updated to March 1975 price levels) was £2684 in provincial medical schools but only £1888 in London medical schools (DHSS, 1976, p. 51). While this paper does not direct itself to the policy issue of whether London teaching hospitals *should* receive an allocation to 'compensate' for lower UGC funding in London, it is clear that factual evidence of the interrelationships of teaching hospital and medical school expenditure is of relevance to those making such decisions. The relevance of the results reported in this paper will be discussed in the final section.

8.2 THE ANALYSIS

8.2.1 Sample and data

The data relate to the years 1969–70 and 1973–4, a separate analysis being carried out for each year. The hospital sample consisted of the thirty-eight Type I acute English teaching hospitals over 100 beds that had medical undergraduates undergoing training.[4] The medical school sample consisted of the twenty English medical schools associated with the thirty-eight hospitals.

Problems exist in the matching of hospital and medical school data. First, only the main acute (Type I) hospitals are considered, and to the extent that clinical teaching is carried out in other hospitals the analysis is incomplete. Second, in most cases one medical school is common to more than one Type I hospital. To avoid making an arbitrary assumption with regard to the extent of interrelationship between the medical school and each Type I hospital in its group, the analysis has been performed twice, first including all associated Type I hospitals and then including just one hospital per medical school. (In the latter case the main teaching hospital was included.)

8.2.2 Procedure

The first stage in the analysis was to define those medical school variables that may have an influence on teaching hospital cost levels. Using data made available by UGC, the following were defined for each of the two years:[5]

(a) General measures of expenditure

$$(SUC_1) - \text{student unit cost} = \frac{\text{total (net) expenditure}}{\text{undergraduate student load}}$$

This is the measure of 'unit cost' often quoted when referring to university departmental expenditure. Another variable to reflect unit cost (SUC_2) was also included:

$$(SUC_2) - \text{student unit cost including specific expenditure} = \frac{\text{total (net) expenditure and other expenditure from specific income}}{\text{undergraduate student load}}$$

(SUC_2) was included because expenditure from specific income[6] varies greatly between medical schools, and the extent to which 'specific' income could substitute for general income was not clear. In the event, (SUC_1) and (SUC_2) did not perform markedly differently in the analysis.

(b) Measures of relative research expenditure

$$(RESRAT) - \text{research ratio} = \frac{\text{expenditure from research grants}}{\text{total (net) expenditure}}$$

$$(RESCAS) - \text{research expenditure per hospital inpatient case} = \frac{\text{expenditure from research grants}}{\text{number of Type I cases}}$$

(c) Measures of staffing and relative expenditure on staff

$$(SALRAT) - \text{salary ratio} = \frac{\text{salaries of teaching and research staff}}{\text{total (net) expenditure}}$$

$$(STASTD) - \text{staff: student ratio} = \frac{\text{number of full-time teaching and research staff}}{\text{undergraduate student load}}$$

$$(WHOFIN) - \text{proportion of staff wholly financed by the university} = \frac{\text{number of full-time staff wholly financed}}{\text{total number of full-time teaching and research staff}}$$

The next stage in the analysis was to explore the simple relationships between these medical school variables and two measures of hospital cost.[7] The latter were:

$$(ACC) - \text{average cost per inpatient case} = \frac{\text{total hospital revenue expenditure}}{\text{no. of discharges and deaths (cases)}}$$

$$(MEDPAY) - \text{medical pay per inpatient case} = \frac{\text{hospital expenditure on medical pay}}{\text{no. of discharges and deaths (cases)}}$$

If lower levels of UGC input do bring about higher levels of teaching hospital cost we would expect many of the medical school variables, especially (SUC_1), (SUC_2) and $(STASTD)$, to be negatively associated with (ACC) and $(MEDPAY)$. In addition, we would expect two of the measures of relative medical school expenditure on staff, $(SALRAT)$ and $(WHOFIN)$, to be negatively associated with $(MEDPAY)$. Conversely, we would expect the two measures of relative medical school research expenditure, $(RESRAT)$ and $(RESCAS)$, to be positively associated with (ACC). Of the two, we would expect $(RESCAS)$ to be the more prominent since it relates medical school research expenditure to hospital case load.

The statistic used to show the relationship between each pair of variables was the zero-order correlation coefficient. This was calculated between (ACC) and $(MEDPAY)$, and the various medical school variables. Calculations were made for both years and for four samples; the sample of all Type I teaching hospitals; the sample of main hospitals alone; the sample of London teaching hospitals alone; the sample of provincial teaching hospitals alone.

Finally, a multiple regression analysis was performed. This represented a more rigorous test of the associations between hospital and medical school expenditure patterns since the associations were explored while standardising for 'known' (hospital) influences on hospital cost.[8] The hospital variables used were those used in the earlier study of teaching hospital cost structure, namely:

$(BEDS)$ – available staffed beds
$(BEDSQ)$ – available staffed beds squared

These two variables take account of the effect of hospital size on hospital cost levels. Significant coefficients for both of these variables would indicate a traditional U-shaped cost curve.

(LOS) – average length of inpatient stay

(OCC) – occupancy fraction

$(THPT)$ – hospital throughput rate in cases per available bed year

These three variables jointly take account of the effect of intensity of use of hospital facilities on hospital cost levels.[9]

$(LOND)$ – London dummy variable

This variable has a value of unity for metropolitan hospitals and zero for others. It was included to pick up all those influences, such as London weightings on staff pay, peculiar to the capital.

$(CMPX)$ – hospital case complexity

$(SPCL)$ – hospital specialisation

These variables were derived from hospital case-flow data using the method devised by Evans and Walker (1972).[10]

(*STDS*) – number of medical undergraduates per hospital inpatient case.

This variable is intended to reflect the quantity of teaching (per case) in each hospital.[11]

The procedure for the multiple regression analysis was as follows. Taking first (*ACC*) and then (*MEDPAY*) as the dependent variable (*y*), ordinary least squares regressions of the following form were run:

$y = f$ (constant term, *STDS, LOS, OCC, LOND, CMPX, SPCL, BEDS, BEDSQ, THPT*).

Each of the medical school variables was in turn added to the basic equation specification. Two things were looked for.

(i) Did the addition of the medical school variable increase the explanatory power of the equation?
(ii) Was the coefficient of the medical school variable statistically significant at the 5 per cent level?

In this way it was hoped to ascertain whether aspects of medical school expenditure could be identified as influences on hospital cost over and above the 'known' hospital influences.

8.2.3 Results

Table 8.1 shows mean values for the seven medical school variables. It can be seen that, as indicated by DHSS (1976), average student unit costs (SUC_1, SUC_2) are lower in London than in the provinces. This is true for both years. The data indicate that one reason for this may be the lower staff:student ratios in London. The ratio of expenditure on salaries to total expenditure, the proportion of wholly financed staff and the ratio of research expenditure to total expenditure are similar for the two groups of schools. Research expenditure averaged over all Type I acute hospital cases is somewhat higher in the provinces.

The results of the simple correlation analysis present an interesting picture. Taking the sample including all teaching hospitals, it can be seen that there are statistically significant (at the 5 per cent level) negative associations both between teaching hospital average cost per case (*ACC*) and the medical school student unit cost (SUC_1, SUC_2), and between (*ACC*) and staff: student ratio (*STASTD*) (table 8.2). That is, where the level of UGC input to medical education is lower, teaching hospital average costs are higher. None of the other medical school variables appear to be strongly associated with (*ACC*). The same overall result is obtained for the sample of main teaching hospitals alone (table 8.3). However, analysis of the split London and provincial samples shows that, while the same overall pattern persists among the provincial schools, it is not maintained within London (tables

TABLE 8.1

Mean values of the medical school variables

Variable	London medical schools		Provincial medical schools	
	1969–70 $N = 12*$	1973–4 $N = 6*$	1969–70 $N = 8*$	1973–4 $N = 7*$
SUC_1 (£)	1127	1516	1839	2217
SUC_2 (£)	1360	2189	2029	2386
RESRAT	0.37	0.53	0.35	0.42
RESCAS	4.27	11.47	8.14	14.98
SALRAT	0.66	0.69	0.65	0.64
STASTD	0.23	0.25	0.48	0.35
WHOFIN	0.73	0.70	0.75	0.74

* N denotes number of medical schools in the sample.

8.4 and 8.5). For the London sample the correlation coefficients for (ACC) with (SUC_1) and (SUC_2) in 1973–4 have the opposite sign, although they are not significant at the 5 per cent level. Also for the London sample, a significant negative association between (ACC) and ($SALRAT$) in 1973–4 was obtained.

The correlations between the medical school variables and ($MEDPAY$), available for 1969–70 only, were in general lower than those for (ACC). This is slightly surprising since it was thought that medical pay might be one component of hospital expenditure sensitive to changes in UGC input, particularly staffing levels ($STASTD$) and method of university staff finance ($WHOFIN$). The results are shown in tables 8.6–8.9. One reason for a lack of association is that ($MEDPAY$) may be sensitive to the number of distinction awards to medical staff in each teaching hospital. These awards can alter clinicians' salaries by large amounts and would not be captured by this analysis.

In summary, the correlation analysis is rather inconclusive. Some associations have been found which lend support to the view that a lower UGC input leads to higher teaching hospital cost levels, but these are not found in all cases. In particular, the negative association of (ACC) with (SUC_1) and (SUC_2) in the whole sample may be misleading. It is already known that there are many possible reasons for teaching hospital costs being higher in London, other than that of lower UGC unit costs. It is possible that (ACC) may be more closely associated with these influences than with (SUC_1) and (SUC_2).

The multiple regression analysis represents one way of resolving some of these issues. Here, rather than simple associations being investigated, the associations between hospital average cost per case and medical pay per case are explored while standardising for the 'known' hospital influences on hospital cost. The results obtained for the full hospital sample (1969–70) are shown in tables 8.10 and 8.11. It can be seen that on no occasion does the addition of a medical school variable to an equation already containing the hospital variables improve the explanatory power of the equation (as measured by adjusted R^2). Also, none of the coefficients of the medical school variables is significantly different from zero at the 5 per cent level. (To be significantly different from zero at the 5 per cent level the absolute value of the coefficient must be approximately twice the size of its standard error, the number quoted in brackets below.)

Correlations with hospital average cost per inpatient case (ACC)

<table>
<tr><td colspan="3" align="center">TABLE 8.2</td><td colspan="3" align="center">TABLE 8.3</td></tr>
<tr><td colspan="3" align="center">*All teaching hospitals*</td><td colspan="3" align="center">*Main teaching hospitals*</td></tr>
<tr><td></td><td colspan="2">Correlation coefficient</td><td></td><td colspan="2">Correlation coefficient</td></tr>
<tr><td></td><td>1969–70</td><td>1973–4</td><td></td><td>1969–70</td><td>1973–4</td></tr>
<tr><td>Variable</td><td>$(N = 38)^*$</td><td>$(N = 21)^*$</td><td>Variable</td><td>$(N = 20)^*$</td><td>$(N = 13)^*$</td></tr>
<tr><td>SUC_1</td><td>−0.56**</td><td>−0.51**</td><td>SUC_1</td><td>−0.54**</td><td>−0.52</td></tr>
<tr><td>SUC_2</td><td>−0.51**</td><td>−0.33</td><td>SUC_2</td><td>−0.47**</td><td>−0.25</td></tr>
<tr><td>$RESRAT$</td><td>0.10</td><td>−0.16</td><td>$RESRAT$</td><td>−0.03</td><td>−0.04</td></tr>
<tr><td>$RESCAS$</td><td>−0.01</td><td>−0.03</td><td>$RESCAS$</td><td>−0.15</td><td>−0.25</td></tr>
<tr><td>$SALRAT$</td><td>0.22</td><td>0.13</td><td>$SALRAT$</td><td>0.31</td><td>0.11</td></tr>
<tr><td>$STASTD$</td><td>−0.60**</td><td>−0.47**</td><td>$STASTD$</td><td>−0.70**</td><td>−0.50</td></tr>
<tr><td>$WHOFIN$</td><td>−0.06</td><td>0.06</td><td>$WHOFIN$</td><td>−0.02</td><td>0.08</td></tr>
</table>

<table>
<tr><td colspan="3" align="center">TABLE 8.4</td><td colspan="3" align="center">TABLE 8.5</td></tr>
<tr><td colspan="3" align="center">*London teaching hospitals*</td><td colspan="3" align="center">*Provincial teaching hospitals*</td></tr>
<tr><td></td><td colspan="2">Correlation coefficient</td><td></td><td colspan="2">Correlation coefficient</td></tr>
<tr><td></td><td>1969–70</td><td>1973–4</td><td></td><td>1969–70</td><td>1973–4</td></tr>
<tr><td>Variable</td><td>$(N = 24)^*$</td><td>$(N = 8)^*$</td><td>Variable</td><td>$(N = 14)^*$</td><td>$(N = 13)^*$</td></tr>
<tr><td>SUC_1</td><td>−0.03</td><td>0.46</td><td>SUC_1</td><td>−0.57**</td><td>−0.51</td></tr>
<tr><td>SUC_2</td><td>−0.06</td><td>0.45</td><td>SUC_2</td><td>−0.57**</td><td>−0.53</td></tr>
<tr><td>$RESRAT$</td><td>0.25</td><td>−0.55</td><td>$RESRAT$</td><td>0.23</td><td>−0.25</td></tr>
<tr><td>$RESCAS$</td><td>−0.10</td><td>−0.34</td><td>$RESCAS$</td><td>0.34</td><td>0.31</td></tr>
<tr><td>$SALRAT$</td><td>0.06</td><td>−0.60**</td><td>$SALRAT$</td><td>0.47</td><td>0.22</td></tr>
<tr><td>$STASTD$</td><td>−0.27</td><td>−0.37</td><td>$STASTD$</td><td>−0.53**</td><td>−0.49</td></tr>
<tr><td>$WHOFIN$</td><td>0.14</td><td>0.49</td><td>$WHOFIN$</td><td>−0.08</td><td>0.19</td></tr>
</table>

* N denotes number of hospitals in each sample
** denotes correlation coefficients significantly different from zero at the 5 per cent level.

Correlations with medical pay per inpatient case (MEDPAY)

TABLE 8.6	TABLE 8.7
All teaching hospitals	*Main teaching hospitals*

Variable	Correlation coefficient 1969–70 ($N = 38$)*	Variable	Correlation coefficient 1969–70 ($N = 20$)*
SUC_1	−0.11	SUC_1	−0.11
SUC_2	−0.08	SUC_2	−0.09
RESRAT	−0.03	RESRAT	−0.18
RESCAS	−0.12	RESCAS	−0.05
SALRAT	−0.08	SALRAT	−0.07
STASTD	0.24	STASTD	−0.32
WHOFIN	−0.07	WHOFIN	−0.11

TABLE 8.8	TABLE 8.9
London teaching hospitals	*Provincial teaching hospitals*

Variable	Correlation coefficient 1969–70 ($N = 24$)*	Variable	Correlation coefficient 1969–70 ($N = 14$)*
SUC_1	0.38	SUC_1	−0.36
SUC_2	0.35	SUC_2	−0.35
RESRAT	−0.05	RESRAT	0.03
RESCAS	−0.18	RESCAS	−0.02
SALRAT	−0.17	SALRAT	0.13
STASTD	−0.15	STASTD	−0.34
WHOFIN	0.02	WHOFIN	−0.23

* N denotes number of hospitals in each sample.

Further regressions were run for the sample of main teaching hospitals alone, and also for the 1973–4 data. These are not shown since the results obtained were substantially the same as those quoted here. Therefore, the multiple regression analysis suggests that it is not possible to establish systematic relationships between (ACC), (MEDPAY) and the medical school variables, while standardising for the hospital influences on hospital cost.[12]

It should be pointed out that, given the small sample size and the aggregate nature of the data, the results of such an analysis cannot be taken as positive proof of a lack of such relationships. After all, some of the 'known' hospital influences on hospital costs did not show up too well in this analysis either. However, it is from these data that decisions about extra 'compensation' for London hospitals have been made, and additional data are unlikely to be available in the near future. In our view it is disappointing that, even given the difficulties with the analysis performed, none of the medical school

TABLE 8.10

Regressions of average cost per case (ACC), 1969–70

Explanatory variables	I	II	III	IV	V	VI	VII	VIII
Constant term	-2.96 (65.25)	-7.21 (66.79)	-9.90 (66.88)	3.36 (65.16)	-7.46 (66.56)	-49.80 (83.13)	-3.29 (74.37)	2.22 (68.20)
STDS	3064 (686.1)	3070 (695.9)	3071 (693.7)	3013 (684.0)	2960 (706.0)	3089 (688.6)	3063 (706.9)	3089 (701.3)
LOS	4.26 (3.79)	5.31 (4.45)	5.31 (4.18)	4.55 (3.78)	4.80 (3.91)	4.12 (3.81)	4.29 (5.07)	4.10 (3.88)
OCC	16.99 (69.27)	-6.68 (86.37)	-3.25 (77.07)	-6.67 (72.00)	0.93 (73.11)	19.99 (69.56)	16.44 (89.76)	19.82 (70.94)
LOND	24.20 (5.78)	22.57 (6.81)	22.59 (6.38)	23.85 (5.76)	25.98 (6.39)	24.62 (5.82)	24.16 (6.75)	23.82 (5.99)
CMPX	-3.69 (11.26)	-1.16 (12.63)	-0.13 (12.72)	0.74 (11.86)	-0.41 (11.94)	-5.19 (11.41)	-3.65 (12.14)	-3.76 (11.45)
SPCL	9.12 (4.73)	8.18 (5.20)	8.00 (5.11)	7.32 (4.98)	8.10 (4.90)	10.04 (4.86)	9.10 (5.03)	9.43 (4.92)
BEDS	0.05 (0.06)	0.05 (0.06)	0.04 (0.07)	0.05 (0.06)	0.05 (0.06)	0.06 (0.06)	0.05 (0.07)	0.05 (0.06)

	(1)	(2)	(3)	(4)	(5)	(6)	(7)	(8)
$BEDSQ$	-0.29×10^{-4} (0.61×10^{-4})	-0.25×10^{-4} (0.62×10^{-4})	-0.24×10^{-4} (0.62×10^{-4})	-0.27×10^{-4} (0.61×10^{-4})	-0.21×10^{-4} (0.62×10^{-4})	-0.38×10^{-4} (0.62×10^{-4})	-0.29×10^{-4} (0.62×10^{-4})	-0.26×10^{-4} (0.63×10^{-4})
$THPT$	0.13 (1.72)	0.75 (2.19)	0.78 (2.02)	0.22 (1.71)	0.39 (1.78)	0.21 (1.73)	0.14 (2.58)	0.06 (1.76)
SUC_1	—	-0.003 (0.006)	—	—	—	—	—	—
SUC_2	—	—	-0.003 (0.005)	—	—	—	—	—
$RESRAT$	—	—	—	20.13 (17.74)	—	—	—	—
$RESCAS$	—	—	—	—	0.56 (0.72)	—	—	—
$SALRAT$	—	—	—	—	—	62.16 (68.02)	—	—
$STASTD$	—	—	—	—	—	—	-0.23 (23.50)	—
$WHOFIN$	—	—	—	—	—	—	—	-5.22 (16.03)
$\bar{R}^2$	0.71	0.70	0.70	0.71	0.70	0.70	0.69	0.69

TABLE 8.11

Regressions of medical pay per case (MEDPAY), 1969–70

Explanatory variables	I	II	III	IV	V	VI	VII	VIII
Constant term	9.38 (7.20)	9.92 (7.36)	10.32 (7.35)	9.38 (7.36)	9.43 (7.36)	15.50 (9.12)	9.87 (8.21)	10.45 (7.49)
STDS	194.2 (75.74)	193.5 (76.72)	193.2 (76.29)	194.2 (7.73)	192.9 (78.08)	191.0 (75.55)	195.8 (78.01)	199.3 (77.03)
LOS	-0.07 (0.42)	-0.21 (0.49)	-0.21 (0.46)	-0.07 (0.43)	-0.07 (0.43)	-0.05 (0.42)	-0.12 (0.56)	-0.10 (0.43)
OCC	0.23 (7.65)	3.25 (9.52)	2.99 (8.48)	0.23 (8.14)	0.19 (8.08)	-0.16 (7.63)	1.05 (9.91)	0.82 (7.79)
LOND	-0.62 (0.64)	-0.41 (0.75)	-0.40 (0.70)	-0.62 (0.65)	-0.65 (0.70)	-0.67 (0.64)	-0.57 (0.74)	-0.70 (0.66)
CMPX	1.26 (1.24)	0.94 (1.39)	0.78 (1.40)	1.26 (1.34)	1.33 (1.32)	1.46 (1.25)	1.20 (1.34)	1.25 (1.26)
SPCL	-0.41 (0.52)	-0.29 (0.57)	-0.26 (0.56)	-0.41 (0.56)	-0.43 (0.54)	-0.53 (0.53)	-0.39 (0.56)	-0.35 (0.54)
BEDS	-0.004 (0.007)	-0.003 (0.007)	-0.003 (0.007)	-0.004 (0.007)	-0.004 (0.007)	-0.005 (0.007)	-0.004 (0.007)	-0.004 (0.007)

	(1)	(2)	(3)	(4)	(5)	(6)	(7)	(8)
BEDSQ	0.68×10^{-5} (0.67×10^{-5})	0.63×10^{-5} (0.69×10^{-5})	0.61×10^{-5} (0.68×10^{-5})	0.68×10^{-5} (0.69×10^{-5})	0.68×10^{-5} (0.68×10^{-5})	0.79×10^{-5} (0.68×10^{-5})	0.68×10^{-5} (0.69×10^{-5})	0.74×10^{-5} (0.69×10^{-5})
THPT	-0.12 (0.19)	-0.20 (0.24)	-0.21 (0.22)	-0.12 (0.19)	-0.12 (0.19)	-0.13 (0.19)	-0.15 (0.28)	-0.13 (0.19)
SUC_1	—	0.36×10^{-3} (0.66×10^{-3})	—	—	—	—	—	—
SUC_2	—	—	0.42×10^{-3} (0.54×10^{-3})	—	—	—	—	—
RESRAT	—	—	—	0.30×10^{-3} (2.00)	—	—	—	—
RESCAS	—	—	—	—	0.005 (0.08)	—	—	—
SALRAT	—	—	—	—	—	-8.12 (7.46)	—	—
STASTD	—	—	—	—	—	—	0.35 (2.59)	—
WHOFIN	—	—	—	—	—	—	—	-1.08 (1.76)
$\bar{R}^2$	0.43	0.41	0.42	0.41	0.41	0.43	0.41	0.41

variables justified their inclusion in the regression equations by increasing explanatory power.

8.3   DISCUSSION

UGC financial provision for the London medical schools is lower per clinical medical student than in the provinces. This has been identified by the recent DHSS Resource Allocation Working Party (DHSS, 1976) as a factor that 'might explain the wide differences in excess costs between London and provincial teaching hospitals', and as one that 'ought to be taken into account in determining the level of SIFT' (DHSS, 1976, p. 51). (The Service Increment for Teaching, SIFT, is an extra revenue allocation to be given to teaching hospitals to enable them to fulfil their teaching responsibilities.)

The empirical work reported here provides little evidence in support of the Resource Allocation Working Party's explanation. There appear to be few consistent associations between medical school expenditure patterns and teaching hospital costs. Some simple associations have been found, in particular the negative association in the whole sample between teaching hospital average cost per case and medical school (clinical medicine) student unit cost (table 8.2). However, this association is *not* found within London (table 8.4). In addition, no systematic relationships can be established between hospital costs and the medical school variables, when these relationships are explored while standardising (through a multiple regression analysis) for the various hospital influences on hospital cost (table 8.10).

It is not the intention here to tackle the policy question of whether the lower level of UGC funding *ought* to be taken into account in determining the level of SIFT for the London teaching hospitals. The question of differential funding between the London hospitals and the others bears on a number of factors. First, this analysis, like the earlier analysis of the costs of teaching and non-teaching hospitals (Culyer *et al.*, 1976a,b), indicates a constant cost uplift (per case) associated with London location. This may or may not be covered by the existing funding arrangements designed to allow for the effect of London weighting (e.g. on staff salaries) (DHSS, 1976, p. 51). Also, case complexity, although not a significant variable in this study of the costs of teaching hospitals alone, was a prominent influence on cost in the earlier analysis. Since it is known that London teaching hospitals treat many of the more complex cases, some of which originate from outside the metropolis, decisions concerning the relative funding of London and provincial teaching hospitals may ultimately involve difficult choices concerning *where* the more complex cases should be treated, and *whether* (given scarcity of resources) they should be given priority over others.

The lack of systematic relationships between medical school expenditure patterns and teaching hospital costs raises other interesting issues, for, if the analysis is correct, London medical schools appear to be producing medical education at lower 'cost'. Although cost comparisons in the university sector were outside the immediate scope of this investigation, we set out possible explanations for such a 'cost' differential below since these indicate areas for future study.

(i) The first explanation lies in the definition of 'cost'. These data refer only to revenue expenditure, so the analysis makes no allowance for differing levels of capital provision. Also, the UGC data refer only to university *departmental* costs, the relative consumption of central resources by clinical medicine departments being excluded.

Another possibility is that others, such as the students themselves or medical staff, may be bearing correspondingly more of the costs of producing medical education in London. For instance, NHS medical staff may give up some of their personal time to be involved in teaching, rather than reducing their NHS workload. Alternatively, the lower staff:student ratios in London may imply less formal class contact time, with students committing more of their own time to learning.

(ii) The second explanation lies in the definition of the 'output' of medical education, which in this analysis is implicitly taken to be the student-year. Lower unit costs could imply lower quality, although there are clearly limits to the extent of this possibility since all medical schools (and their associated teaching hospitals) produce graduates acceptable to the examining bodies. There is, however, little evidence with which we are acquainted to suggest that lower cost teaching technologies do actually reduce the quality of education – indeed, the reverse may be the case.

(iii) Finally, it may be that the very 'joint' or complementary nature of the teaching and treating functions allows those medical staff involved both in educational and therapeutic work to accomplish more work in total at no extra cost. (The same is often said of teaching and research in other academic departments.)

The speculative nature of such explanations suggests that much could be gained from more detailed study of the effectiveness and efficiency of different approaches to the education of medical undergraduates. Our own analysis does no more than set the scene for such further investigations. At the general level it is clear, both from this and from our earlier work, that medical school planning cannot be properly undertaken without a full consideration of the substantial expenditures that it implies for the NHS. More specifically, and of particular relevance in the context of the current debate over the implications of RAWP, the current evidence does not, on closer inspection, necessarily indicate either that the London schools 'need' additional 'topping-up' finance in view of their lower per student UGC funding, or that they are producing second-rate students. It may just be that they are among the most efficient teaching institutions in the country – a

possibility that can be checked only by deeper study of the educational
process in London and elsewhere.

NOTES

1. The authors are grateful to DHSS and UGC for providing data, and to DHSS for
   supporting research into teaching hospital costs at the Institute of Social and Economic
   Research, University of York. This paper is a by-product of a project involving J. Wiseman
   at the University of York and P. A. West at the University of Sussex, whose indirect
   contributions to the present paper are gratefully acknowledged. Finally, the authors are
   indebted to Lionel Needleman who commented on an earlier draft of this paper.
2. For instance, the rehearsing of therapies with students could lead to improved (treatment)
   performance on the part of the teacher. Conversely, the fulfilment of teaching objectives
   may increase the length of hospital stays, and the involvement of students in treatments
   (e.g. ward rounds) could be a source of disutility to some patients.
3. Discussion of efficiency is difficult in both health and education sectors, primarily owing
   to the lack of suitable measures of output. For an approach to output measurement in
   health see Culyer et al. (1971).
4. The hospital sample was reduced from 38 to 21 for 1973–4 since not all hospitals submitted cost returns in that year.
5. All data relate to clinical medicine alone except for 1969–70 expenditure, where UGC
   were unable to provide disaggregated figures (i.e. between pre-clinical medicine, clinical
   medicine and clinical dentistry) for the London schools. It was assumed that each
   London school split its general and research expenditure between pre-clinical and clinical
   sectors in the same ratio as the overall London split. Also, 1970–1 staffing data were used
   instead of 1969–70 as UGC were unable to provide the latter.
6. This is income from grants, etc., which is designated for specific purposes.
7. The choice of (ACC) as the dependent variable raises a number of issues. First, total
   hospital cost was averaged over a unit of output (cases) to reduce the possibility of
   heteroscedasticity and multicollinearity. The problem of heteroscedasticity in the estimation of the total cost function was noted by Feldstein (1967). Upon ordering his
   hospital sample by size (available beds) and calculating the error variance in each
   quartile, he found that the error variances in each quartile differed substantially from
   one another. The problem was not so apparent in the case of the average cost (per
   case) function. The possibility of multicollinearity arises since, in the estimation of the
   total cost function, one would include the number of medical students per hospital as an
   explanatory variable. This is closely related to hospital size for this sample of hospitals.

   Second, the inpatient case is chosen as the unit of output in preference to the inpatient day.
   This is because cost per inpatient day can be a misleading concept. For example, it is
   possible for an institution to lower its average cost per inpatient day merely by
   lengthening patient stays, since the days of care provided towards the end of a patient's
   stay are generally less resource-intensive. Hence a hospital increasing its proportion of
   low-intensity days provided will lower its average cost per inpatient day while
   increasing its average cost per case.

   Finally, it is recognised that the treated case is itself a poor measure of hospital output.
   Unfortunately, no better measure is readily available. For a fuller discussion of this
   problem see Culyer et al. (1976b).
8. These were those factors that had been shown to be systematically related to hospital
   cost levels in an earlier analysis (Culyer et al., 1976a,b). All of them had estimated coefficients significantly different from zero (at the 5 per cent level) in regressions of a sample
   of 260 teaching and non-teaching hospitals. This was taken as a legitimate reason for
   standardising for them in this analysis, although *a priori* one might not expect them to
   perform so well in the regressions of this smaller sample of teaching hospitals alone.

9. In fact these three variables are mathematically related.

$$(THPT) = \frac{\text{cases per year}}{\text{available beds}} = \frac{\text{cases per year}}{\text{occupied beds}} \times \frac{\text{occupied beds}}{\text{available beds}} = \frac{365}{(LOS)} \times (OCC).$$

This being the case, the addition of (say) $(THPT)$ to a regression equation containing (OCC) and (LOS) does not introduce new information. A pragmatic approach to their inclusion has been adopted throughout, i.e. if the addition of the third to an equation already containing the other two improved the explanatory power of the equation (as measured by adjusted R^2), then all three were included. In fact, the effect of these three variables was slight, (LOS) being the most prominent of the three. The coefficients of these variables should not be taken as an indication of the separate cost effect of each.

10. Fuller details of the derivation of $(CMPX)$ and $(SPCL)$ are given in Culyer et al. (1976b). The essential feature of the approach is that those case-types concentrated in a few hospitals are considered more complex than those treated everywhere. A hospital's complexity rating is then derived from the complexity of the case-types that it treats. A hospital's specialisation rating is based on the range of case-types treated. This method of standardisation for case mix was preferred to that of Feldstein (1967) for two reasons. First, it necessitated the inclusion of only two variables (rather than nine) yet gave, in the regressions of the 260 hospital sample, similar explanatory power. (We were particularly keen to reduce the number of explanatory variables used here as the sample size is small.) Second, the Evans and Walker method uses data from all thirty-five hospital specialities.

11. The number of students was averaged over cases since this was considered to be a fairer test of the intensity of teaching activity. While reducing the risk of multicollinearity by using students per case as an explanatory variable (the number of students per hospital is closely related to hospital size), we run the risk of spurious correlation through the regression of ratios (see Brown, 1914). In another part of the work a parallel series of regressions using raw student numbers was run. As there appeared to be little difference in the estimates obtained it was considered that to regress ratios was the lesser of two evils in this case.

12. One complication in interpreting the regression results is that some of the medical school variables are themselves correlated with some of the hospital influences on hospital cost. For instance, (SUC_1) is negatively associated (in the 1969–70 full hospital sample) with (LOS) and $(LOND)$ (correlation coefficients -0.52, -0.53 respectively), and positively associated with $(THPT)$ (correlation coefficient 0.60). Such correlations between regressors could possibly (but not certainly) reduce the probability of obtaining significant coefficients for medical school variables added to an equation already containing the hospital influences on cost as regressors.

REFERENCES

Brown, J. W., Greenwood, M. and Wood, Frances (1914) 'A Study of Index Correlations' *J. Roy. Stat. Soc.* vol. 77, pp. 317–46.

Culyer, A. J., Lavers, R. J. and Williams, A. H. (1971) 'Social Indicators: Health' *Social Trends* vol. 1, no. 2, pp. 31–42.

Culyer, A. J., Wiseman, J., Drummond, M. F. and West, P. A. (1976a) 'What Accounts for the Higher Costs of Teaching Hospitals?' Institute of Social and Economic Research, University of York (mimeo) (forthcoming in *Social and Economic Administration*).

Culyer, A. J., Wiseman, J., Drummond, M. F. and West, P. A. (1976b) 'Joint Costs and Budgeting for English Teaching Hospitals' University of York, Institute of Social and Economic Research (mimeo).

DHSS (1976) *Sharing Resources for Health in England: Report of the Resource Allocation Working Party* London, HMSO.

Evans, R. G. and Walker, H. D. (1972) 'Information Theory and the Analysis of Hospital Cost Structure' *Canadian Journal of Economics* vol. 5, no. 3, pp. 398–418.

Feldstein, M. S. (1967) *Economic Analysis for Health Service Efficiency* Amsterdam, North-Holland.

UGC (1971) *Sharing of Hospital Laboratory Services*, Paper 13/M/71, Medical Sub-Committee, 25 May 1971.

UGC (1975) *Note to the Forum on Financing Medical Education*, Association of the Study of Medical Education, 28 May 1975.

Verry, D. W. and Layard, P. R. G. (1975) 'Cost Functions for University Teaching and Research' *Economic Journal* vol. 85, no. 337, pp. 55–74.

9. Sharing Resources for Health in England – the Case of Teaching Hospitals

M. F. Drummond[1]

9.1 INTRODUCTION

If the proposals of the recent DHSS Resource Allocation Working Party (RAWP) (DHSS, 1976) are implemented, some teaching areas and districts, particularly in London, are likely to experience a shortfall in funds. Under the new plans for revenue allocation there will be a general redistribution away from the metropolitan regions, and in addition teaching areas and districts will be guaranteed funds (in the form of an allowance known as the Service Increment for Teaching, SIFT) to cover only part of the 'excess' cost of teaching hospitals over and above non-teaching hospitals. Most of the London teaching hospitals have excess costs, averaged over the number of students attached, well over the median (of which only 75 per cent will be granted). The only relief for London will be adjustments to SIFT to allow for the London weighting on staff salaries and for the lower UGC input to medical education in London.[2]

Under the RAWP proposals, the extent to which expenditure cuts will be made in the teaching institutions themselves remains a matter for local debate, but the possibility of closure of some teaching hospital services and the 'worsening of morale' in London have already been the subject of much debate in the national press. In addition, the RAWP proposals have given rise to a predictable polarisation of views on the teaching hospital 'problem' (of which the London hospitals represent the extreme example). The *British Medical Journal* (1976a, p. 779) suggested that such a redistribution could mean 'the end of excellence' and bemoaned the fact that 'centre of excellence' appeared to have become a pejorative term (1976b, p. 1280). On the other hand the *Hospital and Health Services Review* (1976, p. 374) suggested that an alternative explanation for the high costs of teaching hospitals is 'scandalous extravagance'.

141

The purpose of this paper is to make a contribution to the debate by:

(i) examining the empirical evidence that could be adduced in support of claims of 'excellence' and 'extravagance' in teaching hospitals;
(ii) suggesting that the polemical notions of 'excellence' and 'extravagance' can be accommodated within the same conceptual framework, that of *economic efficiency*;
(iii) highlighting those issues and implications arising from the RAWP report that are pertinent to the teaching hospital 'problem';
(iv) indicating the further information and analysis that would be required for a formal resolution of the main issues.

In fulfilling this purpose, it is not the intention to question the overall basis of the RAWP proposals or to point to their general implications. For example, neither the egalitarian basis of the proposals nor the formula method of financial allocation (with its attendant 'devolution' of decision-making) is questioned. Nevertheless, comment on a part of the RAWP proposals as they affect teaching hospitals inevitably bears some relevance to the general question of health service revenue allocation.

9.2   'EXCELLENCE' AND 'EXTRAVAGANCE' IN TEACHING HOSPITALS

9.2.1   What are 'excellence' and 'extravagance'?

There are probably nearly as many interpretations of these polemical terms as there are people who use them. References to 'extravagance' generally imply high spending, the suggestion being that in some sense the spending may be mis-directed, or 'unjustified'. In general such claims are likely to be backed up by evidence of high spending without much reference to the *results* of such spending.

References to 'excellence' are not as easy to classify. Sometimes the term is used merely to describe the existence of technological hardware and medical talent of the kind found in London teaching hospitals. That is, it refers to the *inputs* to the treatment process. Alternatively, the term may be used to describe the *processes* of care observed in some teaching hospitals, for instance the range and difficulty of treatments undertaken. Third, the term might be used to describe the results, in terms of medical *outcome*, obtained by those working in teaching hospitals. The outcomes could be immediate, in terms of changes in the health state of patients presently being treated, or they could be more distant, reflecting the contribution to medical knowledge (and hence the contribution to the health of future patients) that teaching hospitals make. Finally, the term could be used to describe the *value* to the community of the outcomes (i.e. benefit) produced by teaching hospitals. Despite these possibilities (of which the third and fourth seem the most attractive), the normal assumption seems to be that 'good' inputs or processes result in 'good' outcomes and that these in turn constitute highly valued benefit.

9.2.2 Evidence of 'excellence'

If excellence is defined as an input concept then plenty of evidence of excellence exists. The London teaching hospitals possess a concentration of medical talent and equipment unequalled in the country. The cost consequences of some of these 'high-quality' inputs appear directly as revenue costs (e.g. the higher salaries paid to more highly qualified staff); others may appear indirectly as the running costs necessarily incurred through the operation of complex equipment.[3]

Evidence of excellence in the *processes* employed by teaching hospitals also exists. A recent study of hospital costs (Culyer *et al.*, 1976a,b) showed that teaching hospitals on average treated cases with a higher 'complexity' rating than those treated by other hospitals.[4] This finding is supported both by common observation and by reports in the media.

Evidence of excellence in the outcomes produced by teaching hospitals is harder to find. This is unfortunate, since performance measurement in terms of outcome (i.e. changes in the patient's health state) is to be preferred to other methods. (It is to be preferred since the most appropriate measure of performance is always the one most closely aligned to the objectives of the organisation.) The lack of evidence of excellence in outcomes is all the more to be regretted since some evidence suggests that what is considered 'good' in the input or process sense may not give rise to 'good' outcomes or vice versa.[5] Evidence of outcome excellence in teaching hospitals is restricted to comparisons of case fatality rates from a limited number of surgical procedures performed in teaching and non-teaching hospitals (Lee *et al.*, 1957; Lipworth *et al.*, 1963; Ashley *et al.*, 1971). However, it would be safe to draw conclusions with regard to performance only if it could be assumed that the populations of patients treated by the two types of hospital studied were equivalent with respect to other factors likely to affect outcome. The study by Ashley *et al.* suggested that it would be unwise to make such an assumption, the regional board hospitals in the study having a higher percentage of unplanned admissions. (The supposition was that unplanned admission means that the patient is probably at higher risk *before* treatment.)

Finally, little or no formal evidence of the benefit (i.e. *value* of outcomes) produced by teaching hospitals exists. The informal impression of those who argue in favour of 'centres of excellence' is (no doubt) that the value of the outcomes produced is very high.[6] However, there has been little formal study in this area[7] and most of the evidence adduced for 'centres of excellence' is concerned with input or process notions.

9.2.3 Evidence of 'extravagance'

Like the evidence used in support of claims of 'excellence', evidence of 'extravagance' exists in varying levels of sophistication. At the lowest level, simple comparisons are made between the average costs of teaching hospitals and those of a comparative sample of non-teaching hospitals (e.g. table 9.1). Even at this simple level one might argue for the superiority of cost *per case* comparisons over those of cost *per inpatient week*. This is because it would be possible for a hospital to lower its average cost per inpatient week merely by lengthening patient stays, since the days of care provided towards the end of a patient's stay are generally less resource-intensive. Hence a hospital increasing its proportion of low-intensity days provided will lower its average cost per inpatient week, while increasing its average cost per case.

TABLE 9.1

Average costs of acute teaching and non-teaching hospitals

Cost year	London teaching hospitals	Provincial teaching hospitals	Non-teaching hospitals
(a) Cost per inpatient week			
1969–70	£80.93	£72.27	£55.70
1970–1	£96.74	£87.84	£66.70
1971–2	£112.25	£99.53	£78.58
1972–3	£129.14	£115.66	£91.54
(b) Cost per inpatient case			
1969–70	£142.56	£105.27	£82.51
1970–1	£168.81	£123.15	£95.22
1971–2	£188.16	£135.58	£108.78
1972–3	£212.66	£159.23	£125.36

Source: Culyer *et al.* (1976a).

A more sophisticated approach to cost comparisons is one that standardises for those aspects of hospital structure or operation that are likely to influence cost levels, e.g. the types of cases treated, hospital size, the intensity of the use of hospital facilities (length of patient stay, occupancy rate, case throughput) hospital location and the teaching function. This was the approach used by Culyer *et al.* (1976a,b) in a study of teaching hospital costs, which subsequently formed the basis for the SIFT allocation.[8] The essence of the approach was to ascertain how much of the observed inter-hospital cost variation could be 'explained' (through a multiple regression analysis) by variables designed to reflect those factors outlined above. The study indicated that approximately 75 per cent of the extra cost per case of teaching hospitals was attributable to the teaching function (modelled by the inclusion of student load per hospital case as a variable), the other 25 per cent being accounted for by differences in other factors such as case complexity, hospital location and length of stay.

Such statistical analyses are invariably incomplete, as there are often factors that are difficult to include in the analysis. In this case, no variable was included to reflect differing quality of care since, although one has reason to suspect that such quality differences exist, there is little formal evidence of them (as we have seen above). It therefore remains a possibility that such quality differences (and other factors) may account for some of the cost differences observed between hospitals. To the extent that these factors are correlated with student numbers, their cost consequences will be attributed to the student variable. Thus, it may be that the SIFT allocation is generous if, as suggested in the RAWP proposals, it is to cover the service costs attributable to teaching *alone*.

More detailed analysis of hospital departmental costs has revealed further information that could be adduced by some as evidence of 'extravagance'. While teaching hospitals in general show higher consumption of department services per case, which can be 'explained' in part by the complexity of cases treated, the level of teaching activity and so on, they also exhibit higher unit costs of provision of departmental services, which in general cannot be thus 'explained'. In turn, a high proportion of the unit cost is attributable to higher staffing costs. These could arise either from teaching hospitals employing proportionately more 'expensive' trained staff, and/or from their having proportionately more staff in total for a given workload. A comparison of average salaries and workloads[9] for five types of staff (nurses, and staff working in pathology, pharmacy, physiotherapy and diagnostic X-ray departments) is shown in tables 9.2 and 9.3. It can be seen that, while average salaries (after allowing for London weighting) are broadly similar, workloads of staff in the London teaching hospitals appear to be consistently the lowest. In addition, these differences in workload could not be 'explained' by those factors that explained the more aggregate cost differences.

9.3 'EXCELLENCE', 'EXTRAVAGANCE' AND THE CONCEPT OF ECONOMIC EFFICIENCY

It can be seen that the evidence that could be adduced to support claims of 'excellence' and 'extravagance' in teaching hospital operation is far from extensive. On the one hand, teaching hospitals may provide higher-quality care; on the other hand, some of the 'excess' costs and lower workloads of staff, particularly in London, remain unexplained. However, more important than the lack of evidence is the fact that notions of 'excellence' and

TABLE 9.2*

Average annual salary

Staff group	London teaching hospitals	Metropolitan RHB hospitals	Provincial RHB hospitals
Nursing incl. learners	£869	£878	£861
excl. learners	£1711	£1626	£1441
Radiography	£1515	£1527	£1324
Pathology	£1488	£1365	£1313
Physiotherapy	£1335	£1326	£1151
Pharmacy	£1471	£1400	£1288

TABLE 9.3*

Average annual workload per worker**

Staff group	London teaching hospitals	Metropolitan RHB hospitals	Provincial RHB hospitals
Nursing (cases)	45.7‡	58.6	59.7
(i.p.ws)	82.0‡	98.9	89.2
Radiography (points)	6054‡	8881	8217
Pathology (wtd. reqs.)	15,670‡	18,023	22,796
Physiotherapy (points)	5842†	8084	8833
Pharmacy (cases)	1815‡	2667	2398
(i.p.ws)	3242†	4517	3615
(O.P.As)	389†	501	820

* All data relate to 1969–70. Each hospital sample consisted of Type I acute hospitals only. The numbers in each sample were: London teaching hospitals (10), metropolitan RHB hospitals (12), provincial RHB hospitals (24). Data were not generally available for provincial teaching hospitals.

** The workload units are given in brackets for each staff group. The number of units per worker per annum is obviously dependent upon assumptions regarding the categories of worker included, the contribution of trainees, etc. These vary for each staff group and are discussed in detail in Culyer, Wiseman and Drummond (1976).

† This value is significantly lower (at the 5 per cent level) than the higher of the non-teaching values.

‡ This value is significantly lower (at the 5 per cent level) than *both* the non-teaching values.

'extravagance' are by themselves unsatisfactory. Whether or not 'excellence' is worthwhile to the community depends upon the costs of attaining it. Whether or not higher spending is to be deplored will depend on the benefits that the community derives from the activities that such spending allows. Thus, when appraising alternatives in health care, one should consider both the value of the resources (inputs) used and the value of the products (outputs) produced. This is the notion implied by the criterion of *economic efficiency*. An efficient hospital would either be producing a given set of treatments using the minimum value of inputs (cost), or be producing the set of treatments that maximises the value (benefit) to the community from the resources at its disposal.

Of the two notions discussed, 'extravagance' is related to the idea of economic efficiency. It hints at inefficiency through suggesting that, where high spending exists, it is not 'justified' by the benefit that the community derives from it. 'Extravagance' (or inefficiency) could imply either that teaching hospitals are employing treatment technologies that are not cost-effective (i.e., the same changes in a patient's health state could be achieved at lower cost), or that the 'wrong' conditions are being treated (i.e., other conditions could be treated in order to bring about a greater social benefit from the resources used).

'Excellence' on the other hand encompasses only part of the notion of efficiency since it gives no explicit consideration to cost, except in the trivial case where high levels of input *imply* excellence.

It is hardly surprising, therefore, that most of the evidence that could be adduced either for or against teaching hospitals leaves the real questions unanswered. If teaching hospitals do produce higher-quality care, how does the cost of teaching hospital technologies compare with the corresponding technologies of non-teaching hospitals? If staff in teaching hospitals do have lower workloads, is this offset by a higher quality (and hence value) of the work that they accomplish? The true answer to the teaching hospital debate is likely to be found only by thorough investigation and comparison of *all* the costs and benefits of teaching hospital and non-teaching hospital treatment practices. It is also worth noting that the relevant costs would include those occurring outside the hospital, e.g. those costs falling on other sectors of the NHS, other public bodies and patients. A review of the state of the art in this kind of work is to be found in Chapter 5 above. This task is hardly likely to be accomplished overnight. However, our knowledge of the teaching hospital 'problem' is more likely to be improved if in the future the case for or against teaching hospitals were couched in terms of economic efficiency rather than in terms of 'excellence' and 'extravagance'.

9.4 THE ISSUES RAISED BY RAWP

Although no data exist at present regarding the efficiency of teaching hospitals, it is nevertheless important to consider the way in which the RAWP proposals deal with the teaching hospital 'problem'.

9.4.1 Is SIFT adequate?

The SIFT allowance is intended to enable the teaching hospitals to fulfil their special teaching role. The identification of the true costs of teaching presents several difficulties, not least those arising from the very inseparability or 'jointness' of the teaching and therapeutic processes. (This problem is discussed more fully in Culyer *et al.*, 1976b.) The approach used to identify the costs attributable to teaching, through the exploration of the systematic relationships between cost levels and the level of teaching activity, can almost certainly be improved upon, although nothing better exists at the moment. It is likely that the incompleteness of the approach (e.g. in the omission of any factors to allow for quality of care) leads to an overestimate rather than an underestimate of the costs of teaching alone. Therefore, if 'the sole purpose of the "allowance"... is to cover the additional service costs incurred by the NHS in providing facilities for the clinical teaching of medical and dental students' (DHSS, 1976, para. 4.4), it is likely to be generous to teaching hospitals.

9.4.2 Do teaching hospitals require additional special allowances?

Other than for the guaranteed SIFT allowance, it is the thesis of the RAWP proposals that teaching hospitals should compete for funds at the local level with other sectors of the health service:

Whilst it may be found convenient, and in many cases highly beneficial, to regard teaching hospitals as natural centres in which to conduct research and provide better standards of care, this ought in our view to continue to be a question of choice to be exercised by Health Authorities in consultation with the other interests concerned. [DHSS, 1976, para. 4.5]

This represents a continuation of the change brought about by the re-organisation of the NHS in 1974. (Previously the boards of governors of teaching hospitals negotiated directly with DHSS.) Would anything be gained by further 'protection' of teaching hospitals from these financial pressures – in the ultimate to guarantee them 100 per cent of their 'excess' costs? In answer to this point it is worth noting that, while no data exist regarding whether teaching hospitals are more or less efficient than others, one can make some predictions of the likely efficiency of institutions in differing environments. Industrial concerns, when operating under competitive conditions, are often *assumed* to be operating efficiently, since they must respond to the pressures (e.g. producing the 'right' products at minimum cost) that such competition brings. However, such pressures are not apparent in the operation of hospitals. Indeed, there are some incentives, such as the kudos to be obtained from the employment of sophisticated medical procedures *per se*, that may be contrary to efficiency. This has led one writer (Evans, 1971) to refer to all hospital costs as 'behavioural' costs, i.e. those merely reflecting the choices of the individuals in the institutions concerned, rather than representing choices necessarily arising from the employment of efficient production processes, as compelled by competition in the market place. Given these *a priori* presumptions, one might argue against more financial 'protection' of teaching hospitals. Much as one can admire the fine work that teaching hospitals accomplish, what possible reason could there be for making the more sophisticated medical treatments immune from competition for resources with the more 'bread and butter' branches of medicine?

One possible argument in favour of 'protection' is that the more complex medical treatments are often undertaken as much for the benefit of future patients as for the benefit of those being treated today. That is, they are undertaken as part of a general research and development programme designed to increase medical knowledge, the presumption being that this investment will benefit the community (in terms of better medical outcomes) in the future.

Since under the RAWP proposals all sectors of the health service will compete at the local level for funds, it would be a likely outcome that teaching hospitals experiencing a shortfall in funds (especially in London) may not be able to treat the same set of cases in the same way as before. (Therefore, it could be argued that the possibilities for developmental work will be less than before.) On the other hand some regions, who are net 'gainers' from RAWP, may have more funds. It will be for them to choose whether or not these are to be spent on the expansion of facilities for the treatment of more complex cases in provincial 'centres of excellence'. The implications of this deserve special attention.

9.4.3 Does the movement of funds away from teaching hospitals (particularly those in London) present any special problems?

One argument often used in favour of 'centres of excellence' is that 'the contribution they make ... extends far beyond their boundaries' (*British Medical Journal*, 1976a, p. 779). There are at least three ways in which 'centres of excellence', particularly those in London, may benefit the rest of the country.

(i) The developmental and research work carried out brings about improvements in medical practice. This knowledge is then given 'free' to other localities.

(ii) Many of us derive a sense of wellbeing from the treatment of others in the London hospitals. (Our wellbeing could arise out of genuine regard for the individual treated, or merely from a sense of national pride in excellence.)

(iii) The London centres, because of their particular technical expertise, treat patients from outside the metropolis who cannot obtain equivalent treatment in their own locality.

The first of these points relates to a general 'free rider' problem in the production of medical knowledge. If the discovery and the improvement of new medical treatments *is* expensive, then some regions (or areas) throughout the country could gain by letting others incur the costs of the development work, 'cashing in' by adopting new practices when the snags have been ironed out. (Incidentally, it is worth remembering that the United Kingdom faces the same problem in respect of the world production of medical knowledge.) It would seem logical that, if the benefits from some of the developmental activities in teaching hospitals (in London or elsewhere) accrue to the country *as a whole*, they should be funded (as indeed many of them already are) from central research funds. Clearly, the answer to this problem lies in having a coherent policy for the funding of medical research. (See, for instance, Black and Pole, 1975.) In principle, the questions of *what* research and *how much* research are themselves amenable to economic appraisal. (The expected benefits to the community could be compared with the costs.) However, problems do exist owing to the inseparability of research and therapeutic functions, and to the fact that the benefits from research occur in the future and are subject to uncertainty. Nevertheless, the community must make a judgement regarding the type and quantity of research that it wants since this investment is obtained at the expense of other treatments in the present. The first stage would be an identification of those aspects of teaching hospital activity that could be legitimately designated 'research' and of whether or not these are, or could be, funded from research funds.

The second point is again part of the general problem of valuation of changes in health state. (This is necessary to decide upon an efficient allocation of health care resources.) It is not a problem *particular* to London, merely that one more often hears of exciting developments in London via the media. For instance, those individuals experiencing a sense of wellbeing when hearing of a bone marrow transplant in London may well experience similar feelings when hearing of an expansion of community care for the elderly in Oldham or Halifax.

The third point has added importance as a result of the devolution of health service decision-making and finance to the local level. If the metropolitan regions are to be made worse off, it would be understandable if they required compensation for the treatment of non-metropolitan patients.[10] In principle, it should be possible to identify the flows of patients and the costs of treating them (although the latter would be no easy task). However, several important issues are raised. First, although it is probable that less funds for London teaching hospitals will mean a cut-back (or at least no expansion) in the provision of care for complex cases, there is no guarantee that more funds for some provincial regions will mean expansion of provision for similar cases in the provinces. Therefore, the RAWP proposals may imply a change not only in the geographical distribution of health care resources but also in the uses to which those resources are put. Second, if provincial regions *do* decide to expand their own teaching hospital complexes, will the same level of excellence[11] be obtained at the same cost? If the London teaching hospitals have become inefficient through years of relatively little financial pressure, then it is conceivable that the provinces could achieve the same excellence at lower cost. However, it is possible that it may cost more in the provinces; e.g., there may be a setup cost associated with higher levels of excellence which has already been incurred in London. Also, it is conceivable that inducements may have to be offered to medical staff to encourage them to leave London. Whether or not the latter is the case would depend on whether excellence itself is the attraction, whether medical staff just prefer living in the South East, or whether living there enables them to enjoy other advantages such as a wider scope for private practice.[12] Finally, it should be remembered that, the more specialised (or complex) the treatment, the lower the likely number of potential patients. If this is the case, the simultaneous development or expansion of centres of excellence by a number of provincial regions may lead *ceteris paribus* to those centres being less well utilised than the restricted number of centres in London. Therefore, equality in health service provision, as embodied in RAWP, can have associated costs; and in the context of this particular point it may be more efficient (if the continuation of the treatment of complex cases is what we want) to leave the centres for this in the South East and to allow other regional authorities to compensate the metropolitan authorities for having their patients treated there.

9.5 CONCLUDING REMARKS

(i) Over the years the debate of the teaching hospital 'problem' has been characterised by claims of 'excellence' and 'extravagance'. The empirical evidence that could be adduced to support such claims has been reviewed in this chapter. It is far from extensive, particularly in support of claims of 'excellence'.

(ii) It has been suggested that a more useful concept to be employed in the teaching hospital debate is that of *economic efficiency*. It has the advantage that the polemical notions of both 'excellence' and 'extravagance' can be accommodated within it. There is no evidence of the comparative efficiency of teaching and non-teaching hospitals. Indeed, it may be more fruitful to pursue the question of efficiency not on a hospital basis, but through the appraisal of the costs and benefits of alternative health treatments or procedures as a whole, since many of the relevant costs and benefits of treatments fall outside the hospital sector. To this end, the need for further analysis is just as great in all sectors of the health service. (A review of the state of the art in the economic appraisal of health care alternatives is given in Chapter 5 above.)

(iii) The RAWP report did not explicitly set out to deal with the question of efficiency – it was concerned more with a method of obtaining a more equitable provision of health care resources in England. However, two aspects of its treatment of teaching hospitals do have an appeal when judged on efficiency grounds. First, it has made an allocation to teaching hospitals based upon the best available estimate of the cost to them of fulfilling their special teaching role. Second, in affording no other 'protection' to teaching hospitals over and above the SIFT allowance, it ensures that all types of health care provided in England must compete for funds in the same way. Although no data of efficiency exist, *a priori* one would argue that this system is more likely to encourage it than one in which teaching hospitals (and the types of treatments that they typically provide) were afforded special privilege. (Nevertheless, there is always the risk that the more sophisticated and spectacular branches of medicine will win a larger share of resources than would be justified on efficiency grounds; hence the need for continuously monitoring the efficiency of *all* treatments and procedures.)

(iv) The possible redistribution of resources away from teaching hospitals, particularly from those in London, means that there may be a shift away from the treatment of the more complex cases. (The extent of this will depend on (a) the extent to which teaching hospitals in regions 'losing' from RAWP are able to win extra resources within their own areas; and (b) the extent to which those regions 'gaining' from RAWP use any extra funds to treat these cases at their own 'centres of excellence'.) Two possible implications should be noted. First, if the treatment of more complex cases provides more opportunities for medical research and development work, then these opportunities may be fewer in the future. Therefore if the community wishes to maintain the same level (and type) of medical research, a revision of funding arrangements for research may be required. (In general, it would be desirable to devise a more coherent policy for the funding of medical research.) Second, if provincial regional authorities do decide to promote excellence, there is the possibility that this excellence may be obtained at a higher cost than the retention of that which may already exist in London; i.e., one may be faced with a trade-off between geographical equality and efficiency.

NOTES

1. This paper draws on both the analysis and the discussions of a team researching into teaching hospital costs at the University of York. The team consisted of A. J. Culyer, J. Wiseman, P. A. West (now University of Sussex) and the author. To that extent the

paper is a joint output. Acknowledgement is made to DHSS who provided financial support for the study of teaching hospital costs.

2. In fact, there is little evidence that a lower UGC input to medical education (as evidenced by lower unit costs per clinical medical student) does bring about higher NHS costs (see Chapter 8 above).

3. The *British Medical Journal* (1976b) made this point succinctly: 'The NHS has one of the largest air-conditioned buildings in London at the new St. Thomas's Hospital; it was not designed to be worked on a shoestring.'

4. The complexity ratings for different case-types were derived on the basis that those cases treated in relatively few hospitals were in general more complex. (This approach to the measurement of hospital case complexity was pioneered by Evans and Walker, 1972.)

5. In a study of 296 patients with urinary tract infection, Brook and Appel (1973) found that quality of care (when judged by process) was rated adequate for only 23.3 per cent of patients. However, when judged by the criterion of outcome, care was found to be of adequate quality for 63.2 per cent of patients.

6. Here we must pose the question of *whose* values. Economists traditionally argue that the valuations of those who receive the benefits of health care should be used. The benefits are not restricted to the recipient of the care. They also accrue to his friends, relatives and other individuals whom he may not even know. (This aspect may be important when judging the output of 'centres of excellence', i.e., how much of a sense of wellbeing do all of us experience when we hear of the prolongation of life, or the restoration to health, of a patient in a London teaching hospital?)

    However, most talk of 'excellence' is by those (usually providers of care) who have greater knowledge of the treatments produced. This clearly needs to be investigated further since at best it suggests that some of us genuinely feel we know what is best for others, or at worst it provides a *carte blanche* for any provider of care to justify his or her own operation.

7. See Rosser and Watts (1972) for an example of some pioneering work.

8. This approach was also used for the analysis reported in Chapter 8 above.

9. The workload measures were derived by relating the units of work accomplished per annum (e.g. for nurses the units of work could be inpatient weeks of care provided) to numbers of staff. For some of the paramedical departments, the units of work given in the hospital cost returns were used (e.g. for pathology the units were weighted requests, and for radiography and physiotherapy the units were points.) It is not intended to put forward these workload measures as an alternative to the more detailed information gained from (say) nursing dependency studies (e.g. Barr *et al.*, 1973 Rhys-Hearn, 1974). However, they do give a broad indication of staff utilisation and have the advantage that they can be derived relatively easily.

10. The general problem of the flow of patients across administrative boundaries is recognised by RAWP (DHSS, 1976, pp. 9–10).

11. Excellence being defined here (appropriately) as an output concept.

12. If inducements are required, whether or not they involve an actual resource cost will depend on the types of inducements offered; e.g., more extensive research facilities would involve a resource cost.

REFERENCES

Ashley, J. S. A., Howlett, A. and Morris, J. N. (1971) 'Case Fatality of Hyperplasia of the Prostate in Two Teaching and Three Regional Board Hospitals' *Lancet* ii, pp. 1308–11.

Barr, A., Moores, B. and Rhys-Hearn, C. (1973) 'A Review of the Various Methods of Measuring the Dependency of Patients on Nursing Staff' *Int. J. Nursing Studies* vol. 10, pp. 195–208.

Black, D. A. K. and Pole, J. D. (1975) 'Priorities in Biomedical Research: Indices of Burden' *Brit. J. Prev. Soc. Med.* vol. 29, no. 4, pp. 222–7.

British Medical Journal (1976a) Editorial, 2 October.

British Medical Journal (1976b) Editorial, 27 November.

Brook, R. H. and Appel, F. A. (1973) 'Quality of Care Assessment: Choosing a Method of Peer Review' *New England Journal of Medicine* June 21, pp. 1323–9.

Culyer, A. J., Wiseman, J. and Drummond, M. F. (1976) 'Teaching Hospital Costs – the Analysis of Hospital Staffing Data', report for DHSS, ISER, University of York (mimeo).

Culyer, A. J., Wiseman, J., Drummond, M. F. and West, P. A. (1976a) 'What Accounts for the Higher Costs of Teaching Hospitals?' forthcoming in *Social and Economic Administration*.

Culyer, A. J., Wiseman, J., Drummond, M. F. and West, P. A. (1976b) 'Joint Costs and Budgeting for English Teaching Hospitals' ISER, University of York (mimeo).

Department of Health and Social Security (1976) *Sharing Resources for Health in England: Report of the Resource Allocation Working Party* London, HMSO.

Evans, R. G. (1971) ' "Behavioural" Cost Functions for Hospitals' *Canadian Journal of Economics* vol. 4, pp. 198–215.

Evans, R. G. and Walker, H. D. (1972) 'Information Theory and the Analysis of Hospital Cost Structure' *Canadian Journal of Economics* vol. 5, no. 3, pp. 398–418.

Hospital and Health Services Review (1976) Editorial, November.

Lee, J. A. H., Morrison, S. L. and Morris, J. N. (1957) 'Fatality from Three Common Surgical Conditions in Teaching and Non-Teaching Hospitals' *Lancet* ii, pp. 785–90.

Lipworth, L., Lee, J. A. H. and Morris, J. N. (1963) 'Case Fatality in Teaching and Non-Teaching Hospitals 1956–59' *Medical Care* vol. 1, no. 2, pp. 71–6.

Rosser, R. M. and Watts, V. C. (1972) 'The Measurement of Hospital Output' *Int. J. Epidemiology* vol. 1, no. 4, pp. 361–8.

Rhys-Hearn, C. (1974) 'Evaluation of Patients' Nursing Needs' (parts 1, 2, 3, and 4) *Nursing Times* 19 and 26 September, 3 and 10 October.

PART IV

Manpower

10. The Morale of NHS Staff

R. J. Lavers[1]

10.1 INTRODUCTION

The purpose of this paper is to offer some constructive observations on the subject of the morale of NHS staff in general and of general practitioners in particular. Morale, in the sense in which it is usually employed in discussions of staff, is defined in the *Oxford English Dictionary* as 'moral condition; conduct or behaviour, especially with regard to confidence, discipline, etc.' It is interesting to observe that the term is typically used of a body of troops. Although NHS staff bear some resemblances to members of the armed forces, they have more freedom to negotiate terms and conditions than the latter, are not subject to a rigid discipline imposed by an authoritarian system (although they are of course often bound by professional norms) and are not normally operating in a situation regarded as a state of emergency. The first contention to be made, therefore, is that the use of the word morale, because of its connotations, may often be unhelpful and tendentious, and that we should not lose sight of the fact that it is used as a shorthand expression to cover matters such as satisfaction, confidence and enthusiasm, which form part of the rewards to staff. Henceforth it will be used as an approximate synonym for 'satisfaction'.

This being so, it might properly be asked why we should be concerned about morale. If the improvement of staff morale could be achieved without cost, then a general utilitarian view, to which most people would subscribe, would suggest that the raising of morale forms an end in itself. Typically, however, improvement in morale is achieved only at a cost, in the form of either increased inputs of resources or a deterioration in conditions for groups of staff or patients whose morale is not raised. (It is often assumed that improvements in staff morale automatically carry with them benefits for patients, but little evidence is proffered in support of this proposition.)

In view of this, it would seem sensible to look at ways of improving morale from the point of view of whether or not they contribute to the general aim of the more efficient reduction or management of ill health, and if so the extent to which they do so.

It should perhaps be emphasised that the view taken here of the appropriate role of the medical professions is by no means universally held: many of the institutions making up the NHS display the characteristics of what has been termed the 'labour-managed firm', which may be expected to have as a principal concern the welfare of its workers, with the interests of its customers or clients entering indirectly. This may occur either via the sense of professional responsibility felt by the workers towards the clients (the so-called 'agency relationship'), or via the ability of the clients to constrain professional freedom by, for example, withdrawing their custom in situations where professional and client interests conflict. In the NHS this second route is by far the less accessible to client interests, so that patients are placed very much in the hands of NHS staff. In contrast to this, the view adopted here of the medical profession and other NHS staff implies a wider social perspective: the objectives of the NHS are taken to relate directly to the welfare of patients (not necessarily as construed by each individual practitioner or other professional person), and the significance of professional morale is thus due to its contribution to better medical outcomes or more satisfactory pastoral care. According to this view, morale is a means rather than an end in itself, and the question as to whether morale is too low (or even too high) may be resolved only by investigating what might happen to patient welfare by raising (or lowering) it. Effects on patient welfare may arise owing to the fact that measures taken to raise morale may consume resources that are no longer available for other purposes or release resources by, for example, making staff willing to work for lower rates of pay than otherwise; and owing to the fact that the state of morale among staff may affect patient welfare directly.

Particular examples of this direct effect of morale on patient welfare are the improvement in terms of speed and accuracy of diagnosis by doctors; the prescription of more appropriate treatment regimes; the more effective relief of anxiety among worried well patients; greater readiness to accept organisational changes which may be shown to be of benefit to patients; and, as an extreme case, the uninterrupted functioning of the health service. In considering improvements in morale as a means to objectives such as these, it is required to establish the sort of factors that contribute to improvements in morale on the one hand, and the link between such improvements and the achievement of objectives on the other. In order to illustrate the general difficulties that accompany this kind of exercise, we now survey some of the research on aspects of morale and their correlates among family practitioners.

10.2   SOME EVIDENCE

It should be emphasised that, apart from the invocation of the assumption that improved staff morale automatically improves patient welfare, it is rarely made clear in studies of morale and job satisfaction why these matters are considered important. As a result, the interpretation of many of the results of such studies is made difficult not only because of the subjectivity of the terms used, but also because it is not clear what (if any) social improvements would result, and at what cost, from raising or lowering levels of satisfaction.

As the authors of a recent survey of the literature on job satisfaction have observed, 'several hundred investigations have shown that in general people say that they are satisfied with their work' (Warr and Wall, 1975, p. 14); and general practitioners, along with other groups of NHS staff, are no exception. The results of a survey of GPs conducted early in 1973 by the Consumers Association, for instance, show that 96 per cent of the respondents enjoyed general practice 'moderately' or 'very much'; and, in answer to a question about whether conditions in general practice had improved or changed for the better or worse over the period 1971–3, 85 per cent felt that conditions had improved or remained the same. As with an earlier study conducted in 1964, on which the survey was based (Cartwright, 1967), some variation was present between doctors in different areas, types of practice and age groups, but on the whole the responses indicated a high level of general satisfaction. Such results, however, enable nothing to be inferred about either contributory factors or the effects on patients, and for evidence on these it is necessary to examine in more detail the sources of job satisfaction.

Even at a more detailed level, however, the results of surveys are often ambiguous and difficult to interpret. In response to a question about aspects of their work that general practitioners particularly enjoy, the 1973 sample previously referred to seemed mostly to find satisfaction in dealing with patients (half of all respondents) and in the varied nature of the work (one-third). Approximately one doctor in every five mentioned the independence they enjoyed, the fact that they were helping people, making use of their specialised skills and gaining a knowledge of families and communities. To offset these sources of enjoyment there were several sources of frustration encountered by the GPs, the most important of which were late calls from patients and the presentation of trivial conditions, each mentioned by almost half the doctors in the sample. Slightly less important as sources of frustration were the difficulty of spending adequate time with each patient (mentioned by two-fifths of the respondents) and inadequate pay (mentioned by one-third). Lack of status in the profession, burdensome paperwork and difficulties encountered with hospitals seem to be relatively unimportant as grounds for dissatisfaction, being mentioned by fewer than one doctor in twelve. The relative importance of these sources of satisfaction and frustration is similar to that observed in the 1964 survey (Cartwright, 1967) and in a further independent sample survey of GPs conducted in 1966 (Mechanic, 1968). Knowledge of these items, however, is still not sufficient for any judgement to be made about the costs of effecting improvements in them or of the consequences of such improvements for the care of patients, and the same might be said about the results of surveys of other groups of NHS staff.

TABLE 10.1

Percentage of consultations estimated trivial

	<10%	10–24%	25–49%	50–74%	75–89%	>90%	No. of doctors
1973	23	32	18	21	6	–	112
1964	15	29	30	19	5	2	420

It is clearly necessary to examine in yet greater detail the attitudes of staff towards particular aspects of job satisfaction, and one such on which information is available is the matter of trivial consultations. That this is regarded as a fairly serious problem by many GPs is indicated by table 10.1, obtained from the 1964 and 1973 surveys, which shows the doctors' estimates of the percentage of all consultations which they regard as trivial. As far as any relevance to policy decisions is concerned, however, this information is of little use owing to the fact that it rests on the interpretation of individual doctors of the word 'trivial', and may therefore be little more than a measure of the variation that exists in what has been called the doctor's apostolic function (Balint, 1968), that is his tendency to define for each patient how he should behave when ill and what he has a right to expect. Even if an explicit definition of 'trivial' is used, such as for instance that used by the Royal College of General Practitioners (1970) ('expected to clear up without treatment within ten days'), the fact that what is regarded as trivial to the doctor does not necessarily seem so to the patient would mean that taking measures designed to reduce the extent of 'trivial' consultations might not be at all desirable in terms of the objective of effectively reassuring the worried well. As one experienced GP has observed, 'the contrast between dramatic illness and triviality is intense, but if the eyes are open, the cases can be equally absorbing' (Lane, 1969).

It is, of course, by no means clear what sort of measures would be appropriate to achieve a reduction in the number of trivial consultations even if this were felt to be desirable. The fact that no clear evidence emerged from the 1973 survey on the relation between doctors' views about the extent of trivial consultations and their use of ancillary staff, and also the persistence through time of the perceived presentation of trivial conditions over a period when team care in general practice has been growing, suggests that the use of ancillary staff has little effect. It seems likely that more scope lies both in educating patients and in educating doctors in ways of dealing with patients. Indeed, many of the GPs in the 1973 sample would concur with this view, since over 80 per cent of them agreed or strongly agreed with the statement that a good GP can train patients not to make unnecessary demands, and fewer than 10 per cent disagreed in any way with this proposition. Similar proportions were found in the 1964 survey (Cartwright, 1967, p. 31).

TABLE 10.2

Percentage of doctors who enjoy general practice

| | Number of patients seen per hour (as estimated by the doctors) | |
	Fewer than 11	12 or more
Very much	69	51
Moderately	29	40
Not very much	2	9
Number of doctors	65	45

A second important aspect on which further information is available relates to the difficulty which many GPs have in spending what they regard as an adequate amount of time with each patient. When the extent to which the doctors sampled in the 1973 survey enjoyed general practice is examined in relation to the estimated number of patients seen in an hour, results such as those in table 10.2 are found. When the estimated number of patients seen in an hour is examined in more detail the percentage of doctors enjoying their work very much drops from 100 per cent of those seeing 3 or 4 per hour to 42 per cent of those seeing 16 to 19 per hour, although those seeing 8 to 11 are more likely (70 per cent of them) than those seeing 5 to 7 (60 per cent) to enjoy their work very much. Ignoring the difficulty caused by the fact that consultation rates were estimated by the doctors themselves, the picture that emerges is that GPs with lower consultation rates enjoy their work more. This picture is further highlighted when the doctors' opinions as to the appropriateness of the average amount of time spent with patients are analysed: just over half of all respondents thought they saw too many patients; and while 70 per cent of those doctors having between five and seven consultations per hour regarded such a number as appropriate, those with more consultations than this increasingly felt that the number of patients seen was excessive. No indication is given by such results, however, of the effect on patients of longer consultations, or of the cost of making longer consultations possible. One way in which longer consultations might be facilitated would be by reducing the size of the list of patients of those doctors above some fixed level, such as the 2000 adopted as the target maximum in the Doctor's Charter of 1965.

On the question of the size of list, the respondents in both the 1964 and 1973 surveys were asked what number of patients they would *ideally* like to look after under their existing practice arrangements, and the distribution of actual and ideal list size are shown in table 10.3. The distributions are

TABLE 10.3

GPs' actual and ideal sizes of list

| | Percentage of doctors with actual list size | | Percentage who think this ideal list size | |
	1964	1973	1964	1973
	%	%	%	%
Under 1500	6	6	8	10
1500 to 1999	9	9	29	39
2000 to 2499	27	33	46	33
2500 to 2999	26	22	14	14
3000 to 3499	} 32	21	} 3	4
3500 or more		9		1

very similar for the two years, but a slight tendency for the mode of both distributions to shift downward towards the mode is evident, particularly for the ideal list size distribution, whose lower mode is presumably indicative of rising expectations among family practitioners. None the less, it is worth noting that, despite the promulgation of 2000 as the target maximum by the Doctor's Charter in 1965, over half the respondents in the survey of 1973 regard a list in excess of this number is ideal. If the question had included some reference to the implications of choosing an ideal list size for resource costs or remuneration, moreover, one might expect even fewer doctors to opt for an ideal list containing fewer than 2000 patients. As far as the resource costs of meeting the target maximum are concerned, the reduction to 200 of the lists of the 85 per cent of doctors in the 1973 sample with more than this number of patients would require 30 per cent more doctors.

Having reviewed some of the evidence relating to morale, the concluding section of this paper attempts to indicate what is required if a more constructive discussion of morale is to take place.

10.3 CONCLUSION

It is clear that, when doctors or any other group of NHS staff are asked open-ended questions about the sources of dissatisfaction, the results are very difficult to interpret in such a way that the implications for any policy follow clearly. The basic reason for this appears to be that individual questions bearing on morale are put *in vacuo*, without reference to the context in which alternative improvements might be adopted or to the nature of those improvements. The consequences are that expectations are encouraged to rise along a number of dimensions and among a host of staff and patient groups, and that no attempt is made to achieve the consistency of expectations between groups or with the available resources. Priority should therefore go to the development of an approach to the analysis of the morale of NHS staff that would make it possible to identify the alternative ways in which morale might be improved, the costs of adopting these alternative means and the consequences for the achievement of the objectives of the NHS of their adoption. An approach similar to this has recently been advocated by the Central Policy Review Staff in their proposals for changes in the joint approach to social policy (*The Times*, 18 January 1977), and one of the chief purposes that their suggestion (for opinion surveys to establish the kind of options that command public support) is designed to fulfil is the avoidance of building false expectations. Similarly, questionnaires might be addressed to groups of NHS staff with a view to eliciting the measures that they regard as desirable if morale is to be maintained or improved, the relative importance of these measures, their costs and their impact on the working of the NHS.

Needless to say, such an exercise would not be easy. Since its chief objective would be the prediction of behaviour (i.e. the choice of a particular morale-raising measure) on the basis of hypothetical attitude statements, one would face severe technical problems such as that of constructing questions having assessable predictive validity and immunity from variations in the environmental conditions familiar to the respondent (Oppenheim, 1968). Previous attempts to predict the behaviour of groups of individuals on the basis of attitudinal variables have in the main been successful in fields where attitudes could be fairly readily compared with actual behaviour, such as the taking up of entitlement to medals (Wilkins, 1948) and the intended size of family (Woolf, 1971). Short of adopting selective experimental methods, it is difficult to see how questionnaires aimed at eliciting preferences with regard to the factors affecting morale could be tested for predictive validity. Such objections, however, apply *a fortiori* to the empirical results relating to morale discussed above, and demands from professional and other groups of NHS staff that are made on the basis of such results need to be vigorously resisted.

NOTE

1. Acknowledgement is made to the Consumers' Association for the donation of the data from their survey of General Practitioners and to the DHSS for financial support which enabled the analysis of the data to be performed.

REFERENCES

Balint, M. (1968) *The Doctor, his Patient and the Illness* London, Tavistock.
Cartwright, A. (1967) *Patients and their Doctors* London, Routledge and Kegan Paul.
Lane, K. (1969) *The Longest Art,* London, Allen and Unwin.
Mechanic, D. (1968) 'General Practice in England and Wales' *Medical Care* vol. VI, no. 3.
Oppenheim, A. N. (1968) *Questionnaire Design and Attitude Measurement* London, Heinemann.
Royal College of General Practitioners (1970) *Present State and Future Needs of General Practice* Reports from General Practice XIII, London, Royal College of General Practitioners.
Warr, P. and Wall, T. (1975) *Work and Well-being* Harmondsworth, Penguin.
Wilkins, L. T. (1948) *Prediction of the Demand for Campaign Stars and Medals* London, Central Office of Information.
Woolf, M. (1971) *Family Intentions* S.S. 408, London, HMSO.

11. Medical Manpower Planning in Britain: A Critical Appraisal

Alan Maynard and Arthur Walker[1]

11.1 INTRODUCTION

The objective of this paper is to appraise critically the attempts that have been made to plan the supply of medical manpower in the United Kingdom in the period 1957–76. Our analysis will be concerned with the history of the forecasts of the supply and demand of physicians and the lessons to be drawn from it.[2] The starting point will be the work of the Willink Committee (Willink Report, 1957), although a brief mention will be made of the Goodenough Committee's (1944) attempt to predict demand and regulate supply to meet this demand. Section 11.2 discusses the rationale of manpower planning in the health field. This is followed by a critical exposition of the planning processes used in the period 1944–77 with which we are concerned. In Section 11.4 there is an examination of the manpower targets set by the official bodies and the extent to which these targets were met. Section 11.5 is concerned with the development of more productive forecasting procedures.

11.2 RATIONALE AND PROBLEMS

The growing interest in manpower planning during the last two decades has been due to the belief that all economies, whether mixed or collective, exhibit shortages and surpluses of different types of manpower and that far-sighted official intervention can mitigate the magnitude of the possible miscalculations. The imbalances between supply and demand are regarded without favour from the individual and the social point of view for a variety of reasons. The individual may suffer wealth losses through 'bad' decisions of his own, and he may also be worse off from the status and morale points of view. Society may be worse off because imbalances in the labour market may have a deleterious effect on economic growth and other macroeconomic objectives as well as on the desired delivery of medical care. These problems are exacerbated by the fact that many types of health care labour are highly specific, so that in times of shortage it is difficult to substitute other factors of production (e.g. less skilled labour) for the labour in short supply, and in times of surplus the unemployed labour possesses skills for which there is little demand in other markets. This specificity problem may be technological (i.e., the health care process requires specific proportions of labour and capital input and these proportions are, at least in the short run, immutable) or institutional (i.e. due to the reluctance of individuals and institutions, such as professional bodies and trade unions, to allow combinations of skills, or skills and other inputs, to be changed).

Imbalances in the labour market arise because of rigidities that restrict the price (wage) and quantity adjustments. Often it is supposed that any imbalances between supply and demand are temporary and will be removed after a short time-lag. For instance, a shortage of a particular skill will lead to bidding by competing employers so that the real wage or salary rate will tend to be increased. In the short run, when the supply of labour is fixed, the higher real wage will equate demand and supply by rationing demand. In the longer term the higher level of remuneration will generate additional supplies of the labour that is in short supply. The wage (salary) system in both the short and long term will, thus, tend to equate supply and demand.

The validity of this standard argument is based evidently on the assumptions that the labour market produces the appropriate price change signals. In the case of the market for physician manpower in Great Britain there are characteristics of the labour market and the market for doctor services which weaken or disturb the adjustment process.

The first problem lies in the organisation of health care in the United Kingdom. The employers (the National Health Service) are the sole buyers of physician services. Medical personnel are themselves organised usually in associations – e.g. the British Medical Association – which are monopoly sellers of the services of their members. Factors such as these on both the demand and supply sides of the market inhibit the workings of the labour market and may make wage/salary movements poor indicators of relative shortages and surpluses – indeed, they frequently prevent relative wage/salary movements from taking place at all, hence tending to perpetuate shortages in, for example, specific specialties of practice such as geriatrics and psychiatric care.

Another problem arising from the labour market for physicians is that the time-lags involved in adjusting the supply of physicians in relation to changes in demand are substantial.[3] The undergraduate education of a physician lasts five years and consists, in general terms, of two years of basic science and three years of clinical work. Graduation is followed by one year (the pre-registration year) of study consisting of six months of internal medicine and six months of surgery. A potential specialist is required normally to do a further six years of training after the pre-registration year. This training period is not formalised and the individual student progresses by applying for appropriate posts. The progression is through the grades of senior house officer (one year), registrar (two years) and senior registrar (two to four years). The training can take place in teaching or non-teaching hospitals and its regional co-ordination is the responsibility of a postgraduate dean in a local university. The Royal Colleges arrange in-training examinations and set qualifying requirements which have to be met prior to examination. Possession of one of these advanced qualifications would appear to be a necessary requirement for advancement in some specialties (e.g. general medicine, general surgery). In practice, the average physician ascends the hospital hierarchy more slowly than may be indicated by this description: the average age of new consultancy appointees is thirty-seven years. General practitioners are recommended to take a further three years' training after the pre-registration year, consisting usually of two years of appropriate hospital work and one year of work in general practice. As a consequence it takes at least twelve years to produce a new specialist physician and nine years to produce a new general practitioner. Substitution between the two groups can take place in a shorter time but the more specialised the physician the more difficult (and costly) is the transition.

In Britain, and indeed in most other developed nations, the length of time required to produce a trained doctor is an institutional datum defended by the medical profession as being in the 'public interest' and not open for negotiation to permit short-run augmentation of the stock of physicians (except perhaps in wartime). The Merrison Report, while admitting the existence of resource constraints, recently proposed to give the profession still greater control over standards of medical practice in Britain by conceding to the profession that general practice was a specialism requiring additional training (rather than a reorganisation of existing training) and by sanctioning the imposition of pre-registration language proficiency tests on immigrant physicians. Power over future standards of medicine is to be given to the elected representatives of all practising physicians.

The possibility of reducing the impact of shortages of physicians, by the substitution of less skilled labour inputs and/or capital for highly trained physicians, is circumscribed also by the restrictive practices of the medical profession – in particular their unwillingness to countenance a thoroughgoing audit of their procedures. This is also a barrier to the achievement of more efficient (cost-effective) outcomes in health care. The absence of a thoroughgoing audit of medical procedures may make it possible in situations of physician surplus to pass the costs of the surplus on to the public by over-doctoring as opposed to redundancy or underemployment.

The foregoing represent some of the limitations on the successful working of the market in respect of physicians. Some of these factors are also obstacles to effective planning. However, manpower planning exercises have been preferred to reliance on imperfect market processes.

The aim of manpower planning in a mixed economy is to predict the future levels of demand for specific types of labour and to suggest how the supply of labour may be tailored to meet these demands. The adjustment of supply as a result of the plan may take forms ranging from rigid official control of flows into the manpower pool to simply providing individuals with better information to enable them to plan their careers. With regard to physicians, planning has taken the form of once-per-decade reviews, producing targets whose realism and accuracy have been conspicuously wanting. It is to these reviews, the way they have gone about their task and the way in which they have influenced policy, that we now turn.

11.3   THE PLANNING PROCESS: ASSUMPTIONS AND PREDICTIONS

In this section we shall examine in detail the activities of the medical manpower planners in the period since the last war. This analysis will be concerned with the assumptions made by the planners and the predictions that were evolved.

The report of the Goodenough Committee (1944) had the virtuous attributes that it was explicit about its assumptions and suitably modest about their validity. Because of the war and the problems inherent in forecasting, the Committee felt that its conclusions had to be tentative. This feeling was particularly evident in the Committee's treatment of supply where it felt that substantial changes in physicians' productivity were likely owing to alterations in the size and structure of practice and in the use of ancillary manpower.

The Committee's methodology was, as they themselves recognised, crude. From data they collected it was estimated that 87.5 per cent of the annual student intake would graduate and that 81.5 per cent of these graduates would work in Britain. These physicians who worked in Britain would represent 91.5 per cent of the annual increment to the physician stock, the remaining 8.5 per cent coming from the Republic of Ireland and elsewhere. Any forecast based on such a methodology is likely to be highly sensitive to changes in the estimated value of the parameters.

After this the forecasts of annual physician stock increments, together with the existing stock, were adjusted to take account of mortality in service and of retirements. Three different assumptions were made about the percentage of physicians in each age–sex group who would remain in active practice – two of these assumptions were hypothetical and assumed more retirements; the third was the actual 1944 figure. On these bases the Committee made various calculations about the number of new medical school entrants per year required alternatively to maintain the existing stock of 45,000, to raise the stock to 50,000 in ten years and to raise the stock to 50,000 in fifteen years.[4] The Committee was cautious in respect of precise policy advice because of the difficulties of forecasting and the sensitivity of their physician stock projections to alternative assumptions. Consequently they proposed only a restricted expansion of medical schools. Notwithstanding the work of the Goodenough Committee, the Government decided to increase the stock of physicians by expanding the annual student intake from the 1942–3 level of 2050 to 2500–600. While the Committee advised caution and slow stock movement, the Government practised stock changes in excess of 20 per cent.

By the mid-1950s the profession was expressing its concern about an excess supply of physicians. Hospital physicians were concerned that there were too many training posts in relation to consultancies. General practitioners were worried because of the fixed-pool system of remuneration, implying that the increasing number of physicians in practice would lower remuneration levels. In 1954 the Cohen Committee on General Practice stated that 'if the rate of entry into general practice continues as at present there will come a time in the not too distant future when the general medical service may be unable to continue to support this expansion.'

As a result of these pressures, the Willink Committee was set up in 1955 'to estimate on a long run basis with due regard to all relevant considerations, the number of medical practitioners, and the consequent intake of medical students required' (para. 1). The Committee's policy advice has been much criticised, and to see why this is so a detailed analysis of the methodology used is necessary.

The first step in the Committee's procedure was to estimate the existing number of active physicians, and to determine the attrition from this stock owing to mortality and retirement. The Committee's independent estimate was that there were 53,260 physicians (44,960 men and 8300 women).[5] The retirement question was discussed in detail because of the fact that after 1958 physicians would, for the first time, become eligible for NHS pensions, and it was thought that some physicians were delaying retirement until that date. The Committee discounted this factor as minor on the grounds that the NHS pension amount available in 1958 would have been small, and instead chose to base their assumptions upon the experience of other white-collar groups. The estimated activity rates of physicians over sixty years of age used by the Willink commissioners are shown in table 11.1. These retirement data were combined with the available mortality statistics to estimate the number of physicians required in future years to maintain the physician stock at its 1955 level.

The next set of calculations involved the forecasting of the likely growth of the various branches of the professions. The Committee considered the possibilities of technological change, which involved changes in the ratios of inputs of physicians to other inputs, but on grounds of its unpredictability decided to make no allowance for such changes in the supply estimation process. Having made this decision, the Committee selected a variety of sectoral targets in an arbitrary manner. With regard to general practice, list

TABLE 11.1

Estimates of physicians expected to be active in each age group over sixty years in 1955 and 1980

	Active men		Active women	
	1955	1980	1955	1980
	%	%	%	%
60–4 years	88	80	60	55
65–9 years	69	35	45	25
70 years and over	37	15	20	10

sizes[6] of 2500 in urban areas and 2000 in rural areas were selected. In the light of this target there was a deficiency of 600 principals in England and Wales and 25 in Scotland in 1955. Hospital staff was divided into two sets: specialists and junior staff. Having considered the hospital building programme (such as it was) and the ageing population, the Committee concluded that a 'reasonable' forecast for specialist staff for the period up to July 1965 was that it would grow in line with the then recent trends at a rate of 160 per year (i.e. at a falling rate). For the period 1965–71 the expansion would fall further to 80 per year. The balance between junior and specialist staff was to be maintained by junior staffing rates growing at the same rate as that for specialists. Further stock additions were required to staff a variety of other bodies but these demands were estimated to be small.[7] The Committee considered it likely that the requirements of the armed forces would fall. The service departments indicated that they wanted their permanent staff to grow from 1020 to 1420, with a replacement requirement of 55 per annum at the latter level. However, short service staff and national service medical officers were to be reduced in number from 1840 to 380. Overall the armed forces requirement was to fall by 1080, and this calculation was of prime importance in persuading the Committee about the likelihood of over-supply.

The effects of structural changes in population were added to these estimates of the levels and trends in demand. The population figures were provided by the government actuary and showed an expected population growth to 1971 of $4\frac{1}{2}$ per cent and an increase of 25 per cent in the number of persons aged sixty-five years and over. This projected change in the age structure led the Committee to argue that a further 75 general practitioners would be needed.

The replacement, expansion and armed forces estimates are shown in the first three rows of table 11.2.[8] The fourth row of this table is concerned with the cross-national boundary migration of physicians. This series of numbers is based on scant empirical evidence. Despite the lack of firm evidence to corroborate any conclusion, the Committee stated with great

TABLE 11.2

Future medical requirements as estimated by the Willink Committee*

	1955–60	1960–5	1965–70	1970–1
Replacement**	1150	1180	1230	1260
Expansion	465	440	280	280
Armed forces	55	55	55	55
Net export	160	110	70	50
Total	1830	1785	1635	1645

* All the data are in terms of annual averages and are mid-year estimates.
** Owing to deaths and retirements.
Source: Willink Committee (1957), para. 107.

confidence that 'there is no doubt that opportunities for doctors from Great
Britain to obtain employment overseas have been diminishing in the recent
past and will continue to do so in the future.' This conclusion was reached
after drawing views from the high commissioners of the Commonwealth
Relations Office, from missionary societies and from the president of the
Medical Registration Council of Ireland. At no point during the decision-
making process was emigration to the United States discussed. However,
it was assumed that opportunities for overseas physicians to practice in the
United Kingdom would decline. On the basis of these calculations it was
estimated that the net export of physicians would decline.

The final element in the estimation calculations concerned the output of
new physicians from the medical schools. It was assumed that the wastage
rates during the medical education process would be 4.78 per cent for male
and 8.45 per cent for female students, and that the level of female students
would remain at the Goodenough level of 20 per cent of the intake. This
led to the conclusion that the annual output of new graduates would average
1855 per annum during the 1955–62 period.

The result of these calculations was a conclusion that there would be a
surplus of 265 physicians during the period 1955–62.[9] The policy implication
drawn by the Committee was that the intake of medical schools should be
cut to 1760 per annum (including overseas students) during the period
1957–70). The medical schools reached the same conclusions as the
Committee before the latter reported and in the autumn of 1957 the medical
school intake was reduced by 10 per cent, bringing the intake rapidly into
line with the Willink recommendations.

Within a short time of the Willink Committee reporting, its assumptions
and policy conclusions were being questioned. The Royal Commission on
Doctors' and Dentists' Remuneration (the Pilkington Report, 1960) argued
in its majority report, like Willink, against the use of remuneration as a policy

instrument in the short run.[10] Furthermore, they argued that the stock of physicians was not in danger of being seriously reduced by emigration, and that the emigration rate was low and adhering to recent trends.

Professor John Jewkes, in his memorandum of dissent to the Pilkington Report, argued, however, in favour of using the remuneration mechanism to affect the supply of physicians, and he put forward the view that the long-run supply of physicians was not as secure as was thought. Jewkes also quoted statistics for the total growth in university intakes for the period 1939–58: 70 per cent for arts, 183 per cent for science, 162 per cent for technology, 93 per cent for dentistry, but only 7 per cent for medicine. Jewkes regarded the last statistic as strangely low. He also called for regular manpower reviews by a standing committee rather than *ad hoc* commissions.

In late 1960 Lafitte and Squire (1960) revised the Willink manpower estimate. While recognising the vulnerability of the assumptions about the quality of care in an affluent society (it may not be unreasonable to expect the physician population ratio to grow with incomes rather than stay constant) and about emigration, the authors chose merely to revise the Willink estimates in the light of changed forecasts of population growth and revised participation figures. They argued that more physicians would leave the labour force at retirement age than had been assumed by Willink. Consequently they argued that 80 per cent of the Willink estimate of the over-sixties in work for the year 1960, two-thirds of the Willink estimate in 1965 and half their estimate in 1970 were more appropriate. The Willink population growth estimate of $4\frac{1}{2}$ per cent for 1955–71 was raised to 8 per cent for the period 1955–70 in line with 1960 population forecasts. Table 11.3 shows the effect of these revisions of the 'requirements' calculations. Instead of the Willink surplus, Lafitte and Squire predicted a shortage of physicians and concluded that medical student numbers should be increased 'from the present 12,000 or so to 15,000'. The Government immediately announced that it had decided to review the data and conclusions of the Willink Report.

The authors of the Platt Report (1961) were appointed to examine the

TABLE 11.3

Future medical requirements as estimated by Lafitte and Squire

	1955–60	1960–5	1965–70
Replacement	1290	1320	1300
Expansion	627	602	491
Armed forces	55	55	55
Net export of physicians	160	110	70
Total	2132	2087	1916

problems of the hospital career structure, particularly the problem of time-expired[11] senior registrars in general medicine, surgery and gynaecology. It was soon recognised, however, by the members of the Working Party that there was a larger, more relevant problem: the provision of intermediate staff for non-teaching hospitals. The Working Party highlighted the fact that not enough British physicians were available to fill the increasing number of available junior hospital posts. To fill the gap between the British supply and the demand for such physicians, an increasing number of overseas physicians were taking up posts in the NHS. Those physicians entering the junior hospital grades were experiencing difficulty in obtaining promotion out of the registrar–senior registrar grades. These blockages were held to have accounted in part for the reluctance of some British physicians to enter the hospital system.

The Platt Working Party proposals maintained the Willink tradition by treating physicians as passive participants in the manpower game. The Working Party argued that physicians intending to go into general practice should be persuaded to spend up to a further two years in hospital work after the completion of their pre-registration year (i.e. after full registration). It was proposed also that a new permanent career grade below the consultant, the medical assistant grade, should be created. Finally, the Working Party proposed that regional hospital boards and boards of governors of the teaching hospitals should review staffing in the light of their report, submitting a report to the Minister with proposals for additional consultant appointments and requirements for posts in the medical assistant grade.[12] These proposals failed to recognise that physicians might actively thwart the planners by migrating overseas instead of filling the newly created posts.

Attention was first drawn to the migration of British physicians by Davison (1961, 1962), when he disputed the Willink Report's conclusions about the brain drain. The debate about the brain drain was continued with contributions from Seale (1962, 1964), Hill (1964) and Abel-Smith and Gales (1964). Seale's figures suggested that emigration was running at a level equivalent to one-third of the annual output of medical schools. Abel-Smith and Gales took a sample of one in twenty of the home list of the General Medical Council for physicians registering between 1925 and 1959 (i.e. a sample of 3590 out of 71,910 new registrations in the period) and concluded that, while the Willink Report had got its estimates approximately correct for the period 1952–4, the estimates of post–1954 trends were too low. For the period 1955–9 Abel-Smith and Gales estimated the equivalent of 20 per cent of newly registered physicians were migrating. The Minister, Enoch Powell, had already argued that the Seale figures were too high and that emigration was running at a level equal to 6 to 7 per cent of the output of newly graduated physicians. The apparent greater accuracy of the Abel-Smith and Gales estimates leads to the conclusion that government planning based on its own estimation may have been of dubious value.

The final area in which the Willink Report was attacked concerned their assumptions about female physician participation rates. Lawrie, Newhouse and Elliott (1966) based their work on two surveys, one by the Medical Women's Federation (MWF) and the other by the Medical Practitioners' Union (MPU). These surveys showed that the overall female physician wastage rate was not as high as had been thought. Lawrie *et al.* argued that the pattern of domestic life and rigid NHS employment habits made it difficult for female physicians with young children to re-enter the labour force. More flexibility in employment patterns could, the authors argued, reduce wastage rates, particularly for those female physicians residing in urban areas.

Within nine years of its publication the corpse of the Willink Report had thus been thoroughly mutilated. Revisions in the predicted population growth rate and hard empirical studies of emigration and female physician participation showed quite clearly that the under-pinning of the Report was highly suspect. The Jewkes proposal for regular manpower forecasting was, however, ignored and 'ad hocery' remained the rule.

The next study of physician needs was carried out by Paige and Jones (1966), who attempted to construct a 'coherent set of projections' for all health and personal social services assuming a rate of growth of national output of 3.5 per cent per annum.[13] Their assessment was that 'a shortage of doctors in 1975 is unavoidable. The maximum training and recruitment programmes that are possible can barely keep pace with population growth over this period and can do little to overcome present shortages' (Paige and Jones, 1966, p. 131).

The Paige and Jones study is in two parts. The first is concerned with estimating supply during the forecast periods up to 1975, 1980 and 1985. The authors based their estimates on the Willink calculations for deaths and retirements. They also assumed that better conditions would reduce the net emigration of physicians to 100 per year: about half the level of the previous decade.

On the demand side it was assumed that the need for hospital physicians would continue to grow at a rate of 2 per cent. They did note, however, that a more expansionary interpretation of the Platt Report would imply a growth rate of 3 to 4 per cent. With regard to general practice it was assumed that increasing numbers of both aged and young people, together with a greater emphasis on the community care of the mentally ill and handi-capped, would inflate the demand for general practitioners. Like Willink, they resorted to assumptions about maximum list sizes with the 1980 ceiling objective being 2500 patients per physician and the average set at 1775.

Applying these familiar manipulations led the authors to conclude that in 1980 the required number of physicians would be 82,000, i.e. a rise of 40 per cent over and above the 1960 stock position. This increase would have improved the physician population ratio by 1 per cent per year. Paige and Jones anticipated that the supply of physicians would be only 73,000 in 1980 and 79,000 in 1985; i.e., they forecast an acute shortage of physicians with a shortfall of 9000 in 1980.

The Todd Report (1968) was concerned with undergraduate and post-graduate medical education as well as with manpower planning. The Commission's initial review of the current supply and demand of physicians led them to the conclusion that an acute physician shortage existed and would worsen in the future. The Report presented two sets of estimates, immediate and long-term needs, and asserted that its calculations were conservative with no allowance being made for improved standards of service 'invariably demanded as living standards generally are improved' or for 'the necessary increases in the time spent by younger doctors in study and relaxation' (para. 321).

The Commission's short-term (1966–75) estimates of demand were based on a population growth rate forecast of 0.8 per cent per annum, and as usual the need for medical services was assumed to vary directly with the projected population size. It was assumed that projected changes in population structure would have little effect on needs. For deaths, retirement and female non-participation, a figure 100 higher than the Willink estimates was used because of the predicted effects of a higher proportion of younger physicians in the labour force and a higher prediction about female participation.[14] The Todd net emigration estimate of 300 per annum was seen as 'a realistic forecast of minimum loss'. In estimating the demand for general practitioners, the Commission chose to calculate the number of principals needed in 1975 by using the lowest principals:population figure ever achieved (1961) – 1:2180. The number of trainee and assistant GPs was estimated by assuming a restoration of the 1953–5 trainee and assistant:principal ratio. This produced requirements of 3250 more principals and 1700 more trainees and assistants during the period 1965–75. For hospital physicians the Commission based its requirements estimates on the data generated by the regional hospital boards as a result of the Platt Report (1961). These data indicated that there was a hospital physician deficit of 4700 in 1965. However, the Todd Report argued that 1500 physicians were needed to bring all areas up to the stock levels of the better endowed regions. The flow of physicians to developing countries was estimated as 130 per annum and all other demands were estimated to be 210 per annum.[15]

On the supply side the Commission argued that no contribution to future needs should be made by increases in the number of immigrant physicians. However, their short-run supply estimates assumed an immigration figure of 250 per annum which, together with a medical school output of new graduates of 2070, made a total supply estimate of 2320.

This supply of 2320 per annum during the short-run period 1966–75 was 1000 less than the estimated demand of 3320 per annum for the same period.[16] Over the ten-year period 1966–75, this implied a deficit of 10,000 physicians.

The Commission was so disturbed by these forecasts that it informed the Government of them prior to its report so that training facilities could be expanded as soon as possible.

The Todd Report's long-term estimates were based largely on the physician:population ratio. The Commission analysed the trend of this ratio during the period 1911–61 and found a remarkable uniformity. Taking as a datum their projected 1975 physician requirements, they found that an exponential curve embodying a growth rate of 1.25 per cent per annum passing through this point would also pass very close to the 1911–61 values for the physician:population ratio. The fact that the 1965 ratio was below this trend line was seen as further evidence of the physician shortage in that year. This discovery of a trend led the Commission to advocate the use of a long-term expansion of at least 1.25 per cent; in the end they thought a growth of about 1.5 per cent per annum was about right. This, together with the additional assumptions that the changing age structure would have only a slight effect on physician requirements, that the net emigration after 1980 would be zero and that the female component of the physician stock would remain constant, led the Commission to arrive at the estimates for 1955–95 given in table 11.4. The implication for graduate output of this estimation of demand is in table 11.5. The figures recommended in the Todd Report were revised in 1970 when specific figures were agreed between the Department of Health and Social Security and the University Grants Committee for the intake of students up to 1979. The final agreed target intake figure for 1979 was 4100, as opposed to the Todd recommendation of 4300 each year for the period 1975–9.[17]

TABLE 11.4

Todd estimates of the long-term demand for physicians, 1955–95

Year	Physician stock	Physicians per 10,000 population
1955*	53,260	10.75
1961**	59,200	11.54
1965†	62,700	11.81
1975‡	(a) 68,100	12.07
	(b) 78,100	13.85
1980	86,700	14.84
1985	96,400	15.90
1990	107,000	16.91
1995	119,800	18.01

*Derived from the Willink Report (1957)

** Derived by the Todd Commission (Todd Report, 1968) from a 10 per cent sample survey adjusted for bias.

† Todd Report (1968) estimate.

‡ Category (a) is the 1975 predicted outcome; category (b) is the Todd short-run 'requirement' to meet 'need'.

Source: Todd Report (1968, Chapter 6 and Appendix 13).

TABLE 11.5

Todd estimates of the need for medical graduates 1965–94

Year	Average annual number of British resident medical graduates needed
1965–74	3100
1975–9	3500
1980–4	3850
1985–9	4250
1990–4	4550

Source: Todd Report (1968, table 4, p. 147).

11.3   OBJECTIVES AND PERFORMANCE

In the preceding section we have surveyed the deliberations of the various attempts by public committees, royal commissions and private individuals to forecast the supply and demand for physicians. In this section our concern is to compare forecasts with actual outcomes. This is not an easy exercise because of the changing bases on which official statistics have been collected.

TABLE 11.6

The forecasts

Year	Willink (require-ments)	Lafitte and Squires (require-ments)	Paige and Jones (require-ments)	Paige and Jones (supply)	Todd (require-ments)	Todd (supply)
1960	56,530	59,435	—	58,300	—	—
1965	60,830	62,445	—	59,900	—	—
1970	62,230	64,900	—	62,400	70,400	—
1975	—	—	—	66,300	78,100	68,100
1980	—	—	82,000	73,000	86,700	—
1985	—	—	—	79,000	96,400	—
1990	—	—	—	—	107,000	—
1995	—	—	—	—	119,800	—

In table 11.6 the various total forecasts are shown. In the first column the Willink estimates show the required physician stock rising to 62,230 in 1970. The Lafitte and Squires estimate for the same year is 64,900. The Paige and Jones study forecast a requirement of 82,000 by 1980, compared with Todd's 86,700. For 1975 the Todd Commission estimated a required stock of 78,100 and a supply of 68,100 – a short-fall of 10,000. Thus it can be seen that similar methodology applied at differing times during the period 1955–68 led to a very different forecast.

TABLE 11.7

Forecast requirements and outcomes: physician stock movements
(hospital doctors and GPs)*

Year	Willink	Paige and Jones	Todd	Actual†
1955	(a) 24,841	—	—	24,216
	(b) —	—	—	20,484
1965	(a) 25,591	—	—	24,260
	(b) 23,684	—	—	24,734
1970	(a) 25,966	—	—	24,458
	(b) 24,484	—	—	29,043
1975	(a) —	—	29,260	26,135
	(b) —	(29,346)**	33,034‡	35,316
1980	(a) —	33,700	—	—
	(b) —	32,400	—	—

 * (a) General practitioners (including trainees and assistants), and
    (b) hospital physicians.
** Estimate based on their assumed annual growth rate of 2 per cent to 1980.
  † Health and Personal Social Services Statistics 1975, and Department of Health
    and Social Security.
  ‡ Based on 1975 actual estimate and Todd additional requirements for 1965–75.

The Willink, Paige and Jones, and Todd forecasts of requirements are compared with the actual outcomes in table 11.7. Each forecast and outcome is divided into two categories, general practitioners and hospital physicians.[18] In all cases the forecasted requirement of general practitioners was greater than the actual supply of general practitioners. Willink forecast figures of 25,591 and 25,966 for 1965 and 1970 and the outcomes were 24,260 and 24,458: 'short-falls' of 1331 and 1408 respectively. The opposite result has occurred in the case of hospital physicians. For this type of physician the outcomes have exceeded the estimates. Thus in 1965 the number of hospital physicians exceeded the Willink forecast by over 1000. The surplus in 1970 was over 4500. Similarly the Todd 1975 forecasts were exceeded by nearly 2300.

Thus our conclusions after comparing forecasts and outcomes is that for general practitioners the outcomes were below the forecasts. In the case of hospital physicians, the growth of their numbers exceeded estimates by, in some cases, large magnitudes. These conclusions are appropriate for each of the reports mentioned in table 11.7.

In table 11.8 the estimates of the various bodies of the supply of medical graduates are given for the period 1955–80. The Willink estimates for 1955–60 and 1960–5 were higher than the actual outcomes by 287 and 750 respectively. By and large the Paige and Jones estimates were exceeded. The Todd estimates of supply for the period 1966–75 have been fulfilled, but the output of medical

TABLE 11.8

Forecasts and outcomes: medical graduates*
(of British origin)

Year	Willink	Lafitte and Squires	Paige and Jones	Todd (supply)	Todd (require-ments)	Actual
1955–9	9,150	10,660	—	—	—	8,863
1960–4	8,925	10,435	—	—	—	8,175
1965–9	8,175	9,580	—	—	—	9,206
1966–70	—	—	9,100	9,570 ⎱	31,000	9,593
1971–5	—	—	10,700	11,120 ⎰		11,182
1976–80	—	—	14,800	15,750	17,500	13,951**

* Each figure is the total for the five-year period.
** Estimated.

schools in the period 1976–80 will be somewhat lower than the figure set by Todd.

It is clear that the forecasters have come to mutually inconsistent results and that final outcomes bear little relation to predictions. The 'shortage' of the Goodenough Committee (1944) was transformed into a 'surplus' by the Willink Committee (1957), which was transformed into a 'shortage' by the Todd Committee (1968), and which by 1977, in conventional forecasting terms, may have been transformed into a 'surplus' (Maynard and Walker, 1977). This 'hog-cycle' of surplus and shortage is due partly to the extremely mechanistic approach invariably taken towards the practice of medicine in Britain. Planners have been mesmerised, for no obviously sound reason, by ratios – ratios that are partly the product of history; ratios that are largely the product of unsystematic thought about 'best' practice; ratios that are aggregated averages themselves; ratios, too, that have been merely plucked from the air. But their procedures have suffered also from another general – and even more fundamental – failure. There has not been a single manpower plan for Britain's health services that has been designed so that it can be tested. While it is true that we have compared forecasts of supply and demand with outcomes, the lack of coincidence between the two is remarkable. The reason is clear: a forecast of 'demand' or 'requirements' will not be realised if policy-makers do not agree about what is 'required'. A forecast of supply may not be realised since such forecasts are themselves often designed to alter supply. The exercises to date have all been, ultimately, quite devoid of independent and objective validation. All that can be done with the present forecasting methods has been done – one 'guestimate' has irregularly been substituted for another. These two key failings of recent forecasting suggest the way in which improvements could be developed.

11.5   FORECASTING THE DEMAND AND SUPPLY OF MEDICAL PRACTITIONERS: TOWARDS AN IMPROVED APPROACH

In this section our concern is to suggest improvements that could be made in forecasting procedures for physicians in the UK National Health Service. Some of the improvements discussed could be implemented in the short term. Some, however, will require a good deal more information-gathering and research. All of these improvements should enable forecasters readily to compare forecasts and outcomes, and to detect reasons for their divergence.

The concern of forecasters is to improve the performance of the market by foreseeing 'shortages' and 'surpluses' before they occur and then to activate instruments of control which, by affecting the demand and supply of physicians, mitigate or avoid labour market imbalances. In what follows we will analyse each side of the labour market separately in an attempt to highlight crucial variables.

First we look at the supply side and the factors that affect the elasticity of supply of physicians, i.e. the responsiveness of the quantity supplied to changes in the wage offered. Then we will look at the demand side and demand elasticities, i.e. the responsiveness of the quantity demanded to changes in the wage offered. In both cases, supply and demand, we emphasise that there is a need for short-term (annual) adjustments to the forecasts and consequent public policy. The present propensity to go in for once-a-decade forecasts appears to us to be a waste of resources.

The stock of physicians is affected by a variety of flows summarised in Figure 11.1. Newly qualified graduates and immigrant physicians form the main inflows to the physician stock. The main outflows are due to death and emigration. The only other important variable affecting supply is the participation rate of physicians, particularly the females and those near retire-

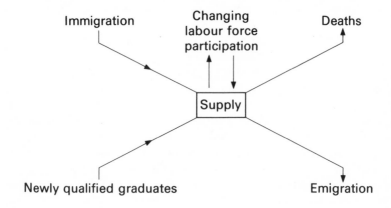

FIGURE 11.1

ment. All these flows can be estimated, and most are amenable to policy variation. Let us discuss each set of flows in turn.

The flow of newly qualified graduates in any particular year is largely determined by the medical school intake six or seven years before. Competition for entry is, at the present time, very intense, partly because of the current depressed state of the labour market for university graduates from non-vocational courses, and partly because of the large lifetime incomes accruing to successful medical students. The medical degree, particularly the clinical component and postgraduate education, has a very high vocational orientation compared with many other university courses. This vocational orientation, plus the dependence for the teaching process on the health care sector for facilities and manpower, makes it attractive to consider the separation of the clinical part of the education process from higher education in general. Such a separation of training into pre- and post-clinical components would add flexibility to the system of producing physicians as some of the output of undergraduate pre-clinical training could be channelled into three-year medical sciences degrees rather than the complete medical practitioner training programme. A development of this nature would make the time-lag between policy changes and policy execution less than it is at present and could reduce the possibility of 'surpluses' and 'shortages' of manpower developing.

Whether greater flexibility is built into the medical school course or not, it is possible to forecast more accurately than at present the output of the schools. Wastage rates should be carefully monitored, and methods other than passing medical school's finals of acquiring registration as physicians (for instance the Conjoint Boards (Maynard and Walker, 1977)), should be explicitly considered by the forecasters. If these things were done it would be possible for forecasters to predict that a given percentage increase in intakes would generate a given number of qualified physicians after so many years. Predictions and outcomes, when compared, would illustrate the efficacy of the forecasters' techniques.

Once the physician has graduated, his participation in the labour force depends on sex, age and the attraction of migration overseas. The retirement age is a mechanism which, when coupled with financial inducements, could be an effective short-term means of changing the number of physicians actively at work. Although postgraduate education is substantial, the skill endowment of physicians may depreciate with age, and consequently their effectiveness may also decline with age. The high level of technical change in medicine may thus make earlier retirement attractive to policy-makers, other things being equal. Clearly, this is a variable that can, with regulation and financial incentive, be used to affect the stock of physicians. The success of such policy instruments depends on the numbers in each particular age cohort and the effects of policy on pension rights. The effects of these variables can be estimated and compared with outcomes, although the estimation must be of a regular nature to take account of inflation and changing relative wages.

The labour force participation of female physicians is a factor that is of increasing importance to forecasters. In 1973 nearly 13.5 per cent of general practitioners and 15.6 per cent of hospital doctors in England were female. In the same year 25.3 per cent of newly qualified physicians (first registrable degree) were female and 31.4 per cent of the new entrants to medical courses were female. Thus the number of female physicians is large and is going to increase in the future. The participation of female physicians in labour market activity will depend on financial arrangements, post-child-rearing training facilities and flexibility in working hours and conditions for physicians who are mothers as well. Once again, the effects of policy manipulation could be estimated and manpower forecasts improved thereby.

The final variable on the supply side is migration, both immigration and emigration. On the immigration side the flow of physicians from less developed countries may be affected by the recent introduction of an examination to test the medical and linguistic competence of doctors with overseas qualifications who wish to practise in Britain. The emigration side of the manpower equation and the immigration of physicians from developed countries, particularly the EEC since the directive permitting the free flow of physicians in the Community, is difficult to analyse. Western Europe and North America have both expanded medical school output considerably (Maynard, 1975a), and job opportunities for potential migrants will be more limited than in the recent past. The 'surplus' of physicians in the European Community may be disinclined to migrate to the United Kingdom because of the relatively lower salaries there. However, the magnitude of the 'surplus' seems likely to be considerable, and consequently a more detailed study of neighbouring physician labour markets is necessary. It must be stated that, even if the total numbers migrating decline, particular specialisms may be disproportionately represented with adverse consequences for the delivery of health care. Once again, regular and careful reviews will enable policy-makers to quantify this portion of the manpower equation more accurately than in the recent past.

The final point we wish to emphasise on the supply side is that the scope for manipulation of remuneration to affect supply is an area of study that deserves greater research input. If salary changes affect lifetime incomes, the relative attractiveness of the medical profession can be influenced. Given imperfect information markets, this earnings information will take time to be disseminated and affect career choice patterns. Obviously, the planning agencies, by publicity, could augment the flow of information. An alternative to remuneration manipulation is the idea that the costs of training should be repaid in part or in whole by physicians. From the equity point of view it is a paradox that society gives medical students a large gift in kind (about £30,000) by training them and then pays them a large lifetime income. The repayment of part or all the training cost would be equitable and the manipulation of the proportion repaid could be used to affect the supply of medical students (Maynard, 1975b). The whole of the financial nexus of training and remuneration cannot be ignored by the forecaster because its manipulation can render useless his work, or, alternatively, provide the means of achieving his targets.

The demand for physicians, and the responsiveness of demand to changing wages and changes in other input prices, is a large area in which relatively little empirical evidence is available in the United Kingdom. We now turn to consider demand in relation to the naive manpower forecasts of the past, and then advocate a long-term policy of reform to take account of the possibilities of substitution between physicians, other labour and capital.

The fact that the previous forecasts have borne little relation to outcomes is not surprising, since generally the planning procedures have involved point estimates and not ranges, or a variety of estimates each conditional on a particular state of the world. For instance, the Willink physician : population ratios depended on point population estimates which turned out to be wrong. Population forecasts are being revised constantly, so the dependence on single population estimates for planning over long time-horizons is foolhardy. For example, consider the fate of the point population estimate used by Todd to estimate 1975 requirements for doctors. In 1966 the estimated population for Great Britain in 1975 was 56.4 million. Instead, the population in 1975 was only 54.4 million, and is now expected to remain constant until the 1980s. This difference of about $3\frac{1}{2}$ per cent between population forecast and population outcome, in a period of less than ten years (1966–75), on the basis of Todd-type calculations reduces the requirements for physicians (physician : population ratio of 1 : 850 approximately) by over 2000 or by rather more than 10 per cent of the total medical school output over the period. Population estimates must be adjusted regularly if forecasts based upon them are to have much meaning.

The usual physician : population demand estimation procedure takes no account of technological change. The Willink Report admitted the existence of technological change but failed to absorb it into the forecasts with any degree of sophistication. Technological change is possible, and hence it is most unfortunate that government inquiries and the private projections have considered physician manpower in isolation from other health service inputs. In 1969 Klarman, writing about the United States, noted 'a tendency to examine requirements for several health occupations at a time, rather than singly' (Klarman, 1969, p. 373). Unfortunately no such tendency has been evident in the United Kingdom.

Estimating the demand for physicians in conjunction with other health professions is sensible because it draws attention to possibilities of factor substitution. The reports discussed in Section 11.3 presume implicitly that such substitution possibilities are limited. But work in the United States, much of it surveyed by Reinhardt (1975), suggests that this is probably not the case. Substitution of other factors (labour and capital) for scarce medical labour offers the possibility of reducing the disruptive effect of physician shortage (if the production and substitution of other factors can take place in less time than the production of a new physician), and it is possible that other combinations of medical input may be more efficient than those to be found at present.

Work on substitution can proceed along two main lines. One line involves the estimation of production functions. With present data limitations, production functions can be estimated only at a fairly aggregated level using crude measures of output (e.g. deaths and discharges) and of inputs (e.g. numbers of staff, numbers of hospital beds). Work of this type has been carried out in Great Britain by Feldstein (1967) and by Lavers and Whynes (1976). A more disaggregated approach similar to that used by Reinhardt (1975) to study physician office practice in the United States could be used if work study data were collected on individual practices or hospital departments. In the longer term the production function approach must be refined by improved measures of output and inputs.

The second possible approach to substitution is by use of the techniques of work study. This approach involves analysis of the tasks performed by the physician to determine whether some of these tasks could be carried out effectively (and efficiently) by other grades of manpower. The efficiency of task delegation must be examined carefully, taking into account not only physician time saved but also any increased patient inconvenience and the cost of any additional facilities required, such as additional treatment rooms.

The two approaches, production functions and work study, could also be used to examine the effects of changes in the organisation of medical practices, e.g. group practice and health centres, on practitioner activity and the activities of related personnel. The policy of amalgamating practices and bringing health professionals under one roof to provide community care appears to have been pursued in the United Kingdom without firm evidence of productivity gains.

Two major obstacles would appear to stand in the way of research, and of the implementation of the findings of such research which might point to the substitution of lower grade labour and capital for physician manpower. The first obstacle is the unwillingness of the medical profession to allow a thoroughgoing audit of their procedures and practices, fearing ultimately an imposition of uniformity of practice in place of clinical freedom (diversity?). A considerable amount of work study has been carried out for lower-grade manpower in the National Health Service but little as yet has been done on physicians. The second obstacle relates to the question of who should bear responsibility for clinical errors made by lower-grade manpower, and perhaps the spectre of malpractice suits against task-delegating physicians or those to whom tasks are delegated.

The physicians' unwillingness to allow an audit of their procedures has wider implications. The official reports discussed in Section 11.2 recognise that manpower requirements could be reduced if productivity could be improved. It seems likely that some large gains could be made by reducing the diversity in methods of practice; the price of clinical freedom at times appears to be too high. For instance, Heasman (1964) found that the length of stay for children over fifteen years old after tonsils and adenoids removal was six days in over 80 per cent of all cases in one hospital group and only one day in 50 per cent of all cases in another group. Morris, Ward and Handyside (1968) analysed the effects of differential hospital discharge patterns for hernia cases. They found no observable difference in the effects of treatment and discharge after one day and treatment and discharge after seven days. Butler and Pearson (1970) have argued that on medical grounds there is evidence that in some cases as many as four out of ten acute patients need not have been hospitalised. Similarly divergences in medical care procedures are observable in general practice.[19]

The implications of these studies are clear. The physicians, in hospitals and general practice, have a wide range of discretion and they use it. As a result of this, and because there is little systematic study of medical procedures, the differences mentioned above are generated. The health care system gives physicians little incentive to compare practices and define the most efficient treatment procedures for varying types of ill health. Even with our present imperfect information, it is apparent that there is a significant degree of inefficiency in the use of resources. If, to take the Morris, Ward and Handyside study, the practice of those hospitals discharging early was adopted by all hospitals, the services of hospital beds and hospital physicians would be freed for other uses. Similarly if Mather's studies (Mather, 1971; Mather et al., 1976) of the comparative medical effectiveness of intensive care and home treatment for some types of heart patient were used as a basis for policy, home treatment would be more intensively used with consequent large savings in beds and personnel and no reduction in the effectiveness of treatment. The Department of Health and Social Security consultative document (1976b) includes a substantial list of published reports on the medical effectiveness of many innovations in clinical practice. Although these studies do not consider the costs, still less the benefits, of different procedures, they represent an important first step in the examination of the work of the physician. The questioning of the efficiency of medical procedures has come from medical (Cochrane, 1972) and non-medical writers (Cooper, 1975; Illich, 1976), and professional power must not be allowed to inhibit this pursuit of greater evidence about the effectiveness of medical procedures.

The research necessary to throw light on the cost effectiveness of alternative therapies, and the possibilities for substituting less expensive factor inputs for physicians, will take a considerable period of time. The evidence that is available at present (e.g. in the Priorities Document – Department of Health and Social Security, 1976a) should be analysed in terms of cost effectiveness (i.e., the equally efficient or more efficient therapies described by these studies should be costed and compared with the costs of alternative therapies) and changes in work practice implemented where appropriate. It is possible that relatively ineffective but cheap types of care may be more cost-effective than more effective but expensive types of care.

The responsiveness of the demand for physician labour to changing rewards may be of increasing importance in the near future. If the medical schools produce the predicted outflow of graduates in the next decade, perhaps the only way in which these people can be absorbed in the labour force is if the real wage of physicians is allowed to decline. The NHS budget constraint and substitution possibilities mean that employment prospects may be bleak unless such a decline is permitted to occur. At the going wage there will be an excess supply of physicians in the United Kingdom by the early 1980s. Their opportunity to brain-drain will be limited and political pressure to employ them at home will be intense.

The preceding paragraphs have attempted to indicate how forecasts could be improved. There is a need too for forecasters to develop a clearer understanding of the nature and magnitude of relevant variables, and how these variables are interrelated. Short-run regular forecasts which make more effective use of the present information stock could improve the relationship between forecasts and outcomes. In the longer run a more efficient examination of substitution possibilities could further improve forecasting performance. The problems are enormous and the solutions are elusive. However the resource costs of 'shortages' and 'surpluses' are such that government agencies will be unable to avoid the temptation to forecast. If there are to be forecasts, the resources could be allocated in a more cost-effective way than they have been up to the present.

In conclusion, there is a variety of ways in which the present forecasting procedures could be improved:

(i)   careful study of the elasticity of supply (i.e. the responsiveness of supply to changing salary and work patterns both at home and abroad) of female physicians, those near retirement and migrants;

(ii) the use of a wider range of policy instruments (e.g. remuneration and flexible, less specific, courses of study) to influence the supply and demand of physicians;

(iii) the use of range, rather than point, estimates for population and physician forecasts;

(iv) greater investigation of substitution possibilities;

(v)   the production of regular annual forecasts showing the cost of alternative policies.

These improvements should be implemented in a way that avoids the failures summarised at the end of the preceding section – use of arbitrary ratios and the practice of forecasting in a manner that prevents testing of the efficacy of the forecasts. Firstly, techniques have to be devised by which it is possible to evaluate ratios. Secondly, plans have to be adjusted to take account of the continuous variability of ratios as time, technology and circumstances vary. Next, the forecasts of requirements should be justified by reference to the ends which physician manpower is seen to be a means and, of course, with reference to alternative means (factor combinations) that are available. Finally, all forecasts of supply should be couched in a way that they are testable: i.e. given policy X, supplies will increase by y. Adherence to manpower policies that follow these rules would lead to forecasts of a more fruitful nature than those of the last thirty-five years.

The degree to which these policies can be carried out in the short run varies considerably. Suffice to say that we believe that far more useful forecasts could be made with the regular and rigorous use of the existing stock of knowledge, although augmentation of that stock of knowledge, particularly with regard to substitution possibilities, would improve the efficiency of forecasts still further.

11.6 CONCLUSION

The performance of the forecasters, when judged by comparing predicted and actual outcomes, has been poor. This inability to forecast with any degree of accuracy calls into question the allocation of scarce resources to apparently fruitless endeavours. However, it is unlikely that the public agencies involved will be able to forgo involvement in such work, and consequently it is to be hoped that their resource-intensive attempts to supplement the workings of the market will be carried out using improved techniques and with greater frequency than has occurred hitherto.

NOTES

1. The authors would like to acknowledge the Social Science Research Council for a programme research grant in Public Sector Studies at the Department of Economics and the Institute of Social and Economic Research in the University of York. They would like to thank Stanley Dennison, David Gullick, Kathleen Jones and Paul Vickers for their comments on an earlier draft of this paper. All property rights in any remaining errors and omissions remain vested in the authors. An earlier version of this paper was published in *Social and Economic Administration*, vol. ii, no. 1, 1977.
2. Throughout this paper we use the term 'physician' to cover all specialties of doctors in the UK. It is hoped that later papers will deal with the manpower planning exercises carried out in the market for nurses and dentists in particular. Please note that throughout this paper we use the term 'physician', not doctor. This is to avoid confusion in non-British areas with personnel holding a PhD.
3. See Blaug (1968), Blaug (1970), and Ahamad and Blaug (1973).
4. Goodenough Committee (1944, Appendix A, pp. 249–57).
5. As the Willink Committee noted, this total was about 2600 greater than that obtained by adding together figures from other sources.

6. The Medical Practices Committee for England and Wales regard areas as 'under-doctored' if the list size is greater than 2500.
7. The Committee assumed that the physician staff of regional hospital boards, the Blood Transfusion Service, mass radiography, private practice and the Medical Research Council would be static. Local authority needs were to be met by filling the 125 existing vacancies; the universities were assumed to require an expansion of 12 per annum; the pharmaceutical industry was assumed likely to absorb a further 50 physicians in the period 1955–60. Thirty vacancies in government departments were to be filled, a further 2 were to be added annually to the stock of government department physicians; and the factory–industry–mines sector was assumed to absorb 45 physicians per annum.
8. Row 2 of table 11.2 is made up initially of 320 hospital physicians, 12 for university posts, 75 for GP posts to cater for the increasing aged population, 45 for industry, factories and mining jobs, $8\frac{1}{2}$ for the pharmaceutical industry, 2 for government departments: a total of $462\frac{1}{2}$. The 465 figure appears to be a round up to the nearest 5 of this aggregate.
9. This 265 is made up of an annual surplus of 25 (medical school output of 1855 minus a requirement (table 11.2) of 1830) during the period 1955–60 and a surplus of 70 during the period 1960–2 (medical school output of 1855 minus a requirement (table 11.2) of 1785).
10. That is, as a means of reducing or increasing the supply of physicians.
11. By 'time expired' we mean that the normal duration of appointment has expired without promotion taking place.
12. These reviews were used by Paige and Jones (1966) and the Todd Report (1968) in their work. See below.
13. The Paige and Jones growth assumptions were optimistic and, in the event, frustrated. For 200 years the UK growth rate has rarely been above the long-run trend, which is about 2 per cent per annum. However, Paige and Jones argued that the lag in altering the supply of professionals was such that the outcomes of the forecasting exercise were not very sensitive to the economic growth assumptions.
14. This is the Medical Practitioners' Union work (see above).
15. For instance, industry.
16. This annual demand was made up, as was indicated in the previous paragraph, of 1350 from wastage and retirement, 300 net emigration to developed countries, 500 for general practice, 830 for hospital service, 130 for service in underdeveloped countries and 210 for other areas.
17. The Todd intake figures for 1965–9, 1970–4, 1975–9, 1980–4 and 1985–9 were 2600, 3500, 4300, 4700 and 5000 respectively. According to their assumptions this implied a graduate outflow for the same periods of 2350, 3150, 3850, 4250 and 4500 respectively.
18. The data in table 11.7 do not sum to the totals in table 11.6 because several sectors in which physicians are employed other than general practice and hospitals are ignored, e.g. local government, industry and central government.
19. See Cooper (1975, Chapter 6 in particular).

REFERENCES

Abel-Smith, B. and Gales, K. (1964) *British Doctors at Home and Abroad* London, G. Bell and Sons.

Ahamad, B. and Blaug, M. (eds) (1973) *The Practice of Manpower Forecasting* Amsterdam, San Francisco and Washington, Jossey Bass-Elsevier.

Beckerman, W. and Associates (1966) *The British Economy in 1975* Cambridge University Press.

Blaug, M. (1968) *Economics of Education* Volume 1, Harmondsworth, Penguin, especially part 4.

Blaug, M. (1970) *An Introduction to the Economics of Education* London, Ailen Lane the Penguin Press.

Buchan, J. C. and Richardson, I. M. (1974) *Time Study of Consultations in General Practice* Scottish Home and Health Department.

Butler, J. R. and Pearson, M. (1970) *Who Goes Home?* London, G. Bell and Sons.

Cochrane, A. L. (1972) *Effectiveness and Efficiency: Random Reflections on Health Services* London, Nuffield Provincial Hospitals Trust.

Cohen Report (1954) *Report of the Committee on General Practice within the N.H.S.* London, HMSO.

Cooper, M. H. (1975) *Rationing Health Care* London, Croom Helm, and the Halsted Press.

Culyer, A. J. and Maynard, A. K. (1970) 'The Costs of Dangerous Drug Legislation in England and Wales' *Medical Care* vol. 8, p. 501.

Culyer, A. J., Williams, A. and Lavers, R. (1972) 'Health Indicators' in Shonfield and Shaw (1972).

Davison, R. H. (1961) 'Medical Emigration: Second Thoughts on the Royal Commission' *Lancet* vol. 1, p. 1107.

Davison, R. H. (1962) 'Medical Emigration to North America' *British Medical Journal* vol. 1, p. 786.

Department of Health and Social Security (1976a) *Priorities for Health and Personal Social Services in England* London, HMSO.

Department of Health and Social Security (1976b) *Prevention and Health: Everybody's Business, A Consultative Document* London, HMSO.

Dollery, R. (1971) in G. McLachlan (ed.) *Challenges for Change* London, Nuffield Provincial Hospitals Trust.

Feldstein, M. S. (1967) *Economic Analysis for Health Service Efficiency*, Amsterdam, North-Holland.

Gish, O. (1971) *Doctor Migration and World Health* London, G. Bell and Sons.

Goodenough Committee (1944) *Report of the Inter-Departmental Committee on Medical Schools* London, Ministry of Health.

Heasman, S. M. A. (1964) 'How Long in Hospital?' *Lancet* vol. 2, p. 539.

Hill, K. R. (1964) 'Medical Manpower, the Need for More Medical Schools' *Lancet* vol. 2, p. 517.

Illich, I. (1976) *Limits to Medicine* London, Marion Boyars.

Klarman, H. E. (1969) 'Economic Aspects of Projecting Requirements for Health Manpower' *Journal of Human Resources* vol. 4, p. 360.

Lafitte, F. and Squire, J. R. (1960) 'Second Thoughts on the Willink Report' *Lancet* vol. 2, p. 538.

Lavers, R. J. and Whynes, D. K. (1976) 'Hospital Production Functions: Final Report' (mimeograph).

Lees, D. S. (1966) *The Economic Consequences of the Professions* London, Institute of Economic Affairs.

Lawrie, J. E., Newhouse, M. L. and Elliott, P. M. (1966) 'The Working Capacity of Women Doctors' *British Medical Journal* vol. 1, p. 409.

Mather, H. G. (1971) 'Acute Myocardial Infarction: Home and Hospital Treatment' *British Medical Journal* vol. 3, p. 334.

Mather, H. G. *et al.* (1976) 'Myocardial Infarction: a Comparison Between Home and Hospital Care for Patients' *British Medical Journal* vol. 2, p. 92.

Maynard, A. (1975a) *Health Care in the European Community* London, Croom Helm.

Maynard, A. (1975b) *Experiment with Choice in Education* London, Institute of Economic Affairs.

Maynard, A. (1976) 'The Containment of Health Care Costs in the United Kingdom', paper presented to a conference at the Fogarty International Centre, National Institutes of Health, Bethesda, Maryland, USA.

Maynard, A. and Tingle, R. (1975) 'The Objectives and Performance of the Mental Health Services in England and Wales in the 1960s' *Journal of Social Policy* vol. 4, p. 151.

Maynard, A. and Walker, A. (1977) 'Too Many Doctors?' *Lloyds Bank Review* July, 125, p. 24.

Merrison Report (1975) *Report of the Committee of Inquiry into the Regulation of the Medical Profession* Cmnd 6018. London, HMSO.

Moore, T. G. (1961) 'The Purpose of Licensing' *Journal of Law and Economics* October, vol. 4, p. 93.

Morris, D., Ward, A. and Handyside, A. J. (1968) 'Early Discharge after Hernia Repair' *Lancet* vol. 1, p. 681.

Paige, D. and Jones, K. (1966) 'Health and Welfare Services in Britain in 1975' in Beckerman and Associates (1966).

Peacock, A. T. and Shannon, J. R. (1968) 'The New Doctors Dilemma' *Lloyds Bank Review* January, p. 36.

Pilkington Report (1960) *Report of the Royal Commission on Doctors and Dentists Remuneration 1957–1960* London, HMSO.

Platt Report (1961) *Report of the Joint Working Party on the Medical Staffing Structure in the Hospital Service* London, HMSO.

Rafferty, J. (ed.) (1974) *Health Manpower and Productivity* Toronto and London, D. C. Heath.

Reinhardt, U. E. (1975) *Physician Productivity and the Demand for Health Manpower* Cambridge, Bollinger.

Royal Society of Medicine and the J. Macy Foundation (1973) *The Greater Medical Profession* London and New York.

Seale, J. R. (1962) 'Medical Emigration from Britain 1930–1961' *British Medical Journal* vol. 1, p. 782.

Seale, J. R. (1964) 'Medical Emigration from G. Britain and Ireland' *British Medical Journal* vol. 1, p. 1173.

Shonfield, A, and Shaw, S. (eds) (1972) *Social Indicators and Social Policy* London, Heinemann.

Sloan, F. A. (1974) 'The Effects of Incentives on Physician Performance' in Rafferty (1974).

Stigler, G. J. (1971) 'The Theory of Regulation' *Bell Journal of Economics and Management Science* vol. 2.

Todd Report (1968) *Royal Commission on Medical Education* Cmnd 3569. London, HMSO.

Williams, A. and Anderson, R. (1975) *Efficiency in the Social Services* Oxford, Basil Blackwell.

Willink Report (1957) *Report of the Committee to Consider the Future Numbers of Medical Practitioners and the Appropriate Intake of Medical Students* London, HMSO.

Wiseman, J. (1973) 'The Greater Medical Profession: Economic Consequences' in Royal Society of Medicine and Macy Foundation (1973).

World Health Organisation (1974) *Graduate Medical Education in the European Region* (Euro 6301 (1)). Copenhagen, Regional Office for Europe.